A CURIOUS WOMAN'S

# Guide to Urology

## UTIs, Wet Pants, Stones, and More!

**DR. STEPHEN F LIEBERMAN, M.D.**

# A CURIOUS WOMAN'S GUIDE TO UROLOGY

*UTIs, Wet Pants, Stones, and More!*

This book contains evidence based facts, as well as ideas and opinions of its author. It is intended to provide general information to enable readers to have an informed discussion with their health care provider(s) in the spirit of "shared decision making". It is not a substitute for medical advice. The reader should and must rely on the advice and recommendations from their personal professional health care provider(s), and use this book to understand those recommendations better. The publisher and author therefore disclaims all responsibility for any loss, risk, or liability, which may be incurred either directly or indirectly as a consequence of any of the contents within this book.

**Veru Montanum Press**

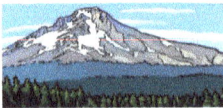

Portland, Oregon, USA 97035

Book cover design by: Susan Bein
Illustrations by: Mogumash
Book layout design by: Saqib_arshad

Printed in the United States of America

stephenliebermanmd.com

*For my mom and dad,*
*Bernice and Eddie*

# What other's are saying about
## *The Curious Woman's Guide to Urology*

*"Dr Steve Lieberman provides straight, unbiased information for common men's conditions that is easy to read and understand. It's a great resource I recommend to my patients and colleagues."*

- Ron Loo, M.D. Chief Emeritus Southern California Kaiser Permanente Medical Group.

*"This is a remarkably lucid, beautifully written discussion of all aspects of male urological medical and emotional topics. Anyone reading this book will be well-informed, empowered, and able to engage in a meaningful discussion with his urologist. Dr. Lieberman explains issues in a tremendously helpful, clear manner, with equal amounts of knowledge, sound advice and charm."*

—Roger Porter, Professor of English, Emeritus, Reed College

*"Looking for a good read on some delicate, sometimes embarrassing topics? You've found it!"*

—John M. Barry, M.D., Professor of Urology, Professor of Surgery, Division of Abdominal Organ Transplantation, Oregon Health & Science University, Portland, Oregon

*"Dr. Lieberman is one of the finest clinicians and passionate teachers about everything related to urology. Whether you are a patient or clinician, this book is packed with useful information about the urinary system. You'll get easy-to-understand answers to the questions you were too afraid to ask. His practical and insightful pearls taught in a conversational style will keep you engaged."*

—Jill Einstein, M.D., Senior Director, MAVEN Project

# TABLE OF CONTENTS

INTRODUCTION                                                    1

CHAPTER 1: Your Body's Plumbing                                 9

CHAPTER 2: I'm Peeing Blood!                                    17

CHAPTER 3: Incontinence and Overactive Bladder                 35

CHAPTER 4: Urinary Tract Infections                            59

CHAPTER 5: Everybody Must Get Stones                           73

CHAPTER 6: Bladder Cancer                                      103

CHAPTER 7: Kidney Tumors, Cysts, and Masses                   123

CHAPTER 8: Emergencies and Trauma                             137

CONCLUSION                                                     143

APPENDIX I: Glossary                                           147

APPENDIX II: References and Sources                            167

INDEX                                                          171

ACKNOWLEDGEMENTS                                               177

# INTRODUCTION

If you're reading this book, chances are you or someone you love has a health problem related to the urinary tract system. There is a lot going on in that system which is comprised of our kidneys, adrenal glands, ureter, bladder and urethra. Most of us don't think much about our urinary tract until something goes wrong—then we want medical help, and we want it quickly. That's because our health—and our peace of mind—depends on having an efficient fluid waste system for everything we eat and drink. When our plumbing gets stopped up or there's a leak in the system, something is wrong.

Most people think urology is a specialty for men patients only. It is for some urologists, but for most general urologists, it's not the case. In my general urology practice, I would say that 30-40% of my patients were women, 40-50% were men, and the rest were children of both sexes.

So I've helped a lot of women with their urinary tract issues, and in this book I go over the many concerns women have brought to me over the years. I'm the guy many came to when they want to know what it is that's wrong, and how to make it right. I practiced general urology at Kaiser Permanente in Portland, Oregon for 31 years. I was

Chief of the Urology Department for 27 of those 31 years. I witnessed remarkable changes in the profession over those decades as advances in medicine and new technological innovations provided a range of options for patients, often options which saved their lives when just a few years before their lives would have been cut short. Yet with our rapidly expanding medical knowledge, technologies and medicines, come not only choices for our patients, but decisions to be made. For every option, there are many considerations, and not everything in medicine is certain. What might work for one patient may not work for another. What one patient can adapt to, another may be unable or unwilling to consider. Whether it's medication, surgery, diet, radiation, or time—the wait and see approach—it's important that you be as informed as possible so that you can make the decision that's best for you—and hopefully, in agreement with your physician.

I've written this book to help you to do just that—to understand your body, particularly your urinary and genital system, better. What does it mean when one or more components of your urinary tract system aren't working properly? What are your options to make it better? What are the risks of the treatment? Knowing these things will enable you to engage in shared decision making—the foundation of not just my approach to medicine, but the recommended approach by all governing specialty boards and anyone who wants to provide the best care for their patients. Shared decision making is a popular concept in contemporary medicine that refers to a decision making process in which both the patient and his or her physician work together in designing the best plan of care for the patient.

This process departs from the traditional top-down model of medical care where the physician tells the patient what s/he needs to do. In shared decision making, the patient's values, cultural background, goals and concerns are considered. The patient (and family) are active participants throughout diagnosis and treatment. By "active participant," I don't just mean the patient shows up for tests and procedures—of course you're going to participate in your own health care by showing up. What I mean is you are armed with information about the procedures, the tests, the medications, and your health conditions, so that the decisions you make are informed ones. By knowing more about your health condition, by being aware of the medications, technologies, procedures and treatment plans available to you, and their risks and benefits, you are better able to ask questions, share your concerns, and work constructively with your physician in treating your health conditions.

We weren't taught shared decision making in medical school when I was a medical student 40 years ago. In those days, such an approach would come under the umbrella of "the art of medicine" or "bedside manner." Some might call it physician empathy. Only recently has the value of patient centered medicine and shared decision making been recognized by the medical profession. Early in my career, however, many of us intuitively appreciated how important it is that our patients be as informed and engaged in their treatment as possible. In more recent years, the increased focus on shared decision making or patient engagement has enhanced and improved the overall care of the patient.

Shared decision making is not for everyone, nor does it apply to every situation or every medical decision. There are some patients who are more comfortable with a paternalistic model. These patients come to me saying something along the lines of "Just fix it doc, do what you think is best." And there are some situations (emergencies for example) in which there is only one way of taking care of the immediate problem, regardless of what the patient might prefer. In these cases, a decision can't be contemplated or delayed without putting the patient's life or organ at risk.

Shared decision making is best suited for complicated illnesses and treatments. Shared decision making is beneficial and well suited for those problems that aren't "fixed" with one solution but will instead require a series of treatments, or for those problems that do not have a single answer but have instead, multiple options, each with risks and benefits. The treatment of kidney stones is a good example where there are many treatment options ranging from active surveillance (waiting for the stone to pass) to minimally invasive to significantly invasive and requiring surgery. They can all produce good long-term outcomes, with only slight differences in "cure rates," but each treatment differs in terms of potential complications and side effects. There is no "one size fits all" treatment for any disorder or disease, so if you are suffering from any urological issue, you will want to know as much as possible about your options, and about your specific disorder, whether stones, a UTI, cancer or other disease.

That's why I've written this book—to give you the basic knowledge of your urinary tract system, the most common problems that urologists treat, and the most effective and up to date treatment options. You're unlikely to need or want to read this book in its entirety, although I encourage you to do so. By having a solid understanding of your entire urinary tract system, you will better understand how the differing components of that system work together. At the very least, I urge you to begin the book by reading

Chapter 1, "Your Body's Plumbing." That chapter is a concise overview of how we're plumbed, and what happens when our plumbing is damaged. Other chapters are organized around various ailments (cancers of urinary tract organs, stones, blood in the urine, infections) or other pertinent concerns (such as urinary tract trauma and emergencies).

In Chapter 2, "I'm Peeing Blood," the focus is on what happens when you have blood in the urine. Because blood in the urine is often a sign of other problems, such as kidney stones or bladder cancer, you may come to this chapter not knowing what is wrong, or you may already know and find that this chapter, along with one or more others specific to your health problem, are valuable reading.

Chapter 3, "Incontinence and Overactive Bladder," provides an overview of the multiple causes of these unpleasant conditions, surgical and nonsurgical treatment options, and daily management of the disorder.

Chapter 4, "Urinary Tract Infections" discusses a relatively common problem for women. In this chapter, I discuss a number of different UTI's, including cystitis, pyelonephritis, and bacteriuria, how each is diagnosed, and how each is treated.

In Chapter 5, I turn to the kidneys in the chapter titled, "Everybody Must Get Stones." If you've ever had a kidney stone, you know it can produce indescribable pain. Kidney stone pain or renal colic has been compared to childbirth. It may take hours, if not days, to pass those cursed stones. For some people, kidney stones are a frequent occurrence, while for others, they appear only once never to return—or they may not cause renal colic at all but present as a UTI or blood in the urine. In this chapter I dispel the many myths you may see on the internet about stones, and explain just how diet, heredity, and other factors lead to different types of stones and how to hopefully prevent them from recurring.

In Chapter 6, "Bladder Cancer," I discuss this relatively common, but mostly curable disease, the many forms of bladder cancer, your treatment options if you are diagnosed with it, and your quality of life should you have to have your bladder removed—I assure you, a cystectomy, the surgical removal of the bladder, does not by any means suggest your quality of life will suffer in any meaningful way, but it may well save your life).

Kidney masses are discussed in Chapter 7, "Kidney Tumors, Cysts, and Masses." I discuss what those lumps and tumors might be, which ones are benign, which are malignant, and depending on the diagnosis, what your treatment options are. The good news is, we've never before had the remarkable technologies that we have today to treat cancers of the kidney. You'll learn which kidney masses are benign and don't need treatment. But, if the tumor is cancer, I'll present the most effective technologies now available.

Finally, Chapter 8 focuses on "Emergencies and Traumas." These are the sorts of things that you probably won't have time to look up beforehand, but may have questions about after you've received treatment, such as injuries, unexpected and life-endangering medical emergencies, or complications related to prior procedures. This is the only chapter where shared decision making is sometimes not possible, because the main concern is saving your life and/or addressing the issue quickly is paramount. I hope you never have need of this chapter, but should you have such an emergency or trauma, I want you to rest assured your concerns are answered.

Regardless of whether you read the whole book or only the chapters of most concern to you, I encourage you to read the Conclusion, where I summarize the importance of good urinary tract health and what you can do to ensure yours is the best it can be. One of those things is knowing how to work with your physician and medical team to remain an informed and engaged participant in your treatment from the very first day you walk into your physician's office. To help you stay engaged, I've included a list of resources, with a link to my website where you can stay up-to-date on the most recent advances in urological care, as well as a Glossary for those terms you might forget after my initial definition.

In closing, a few words on my own personal bias. We live in an amazing age, where information on any topic imaginable is available to almost anyone with a laptop and access to Google. But with that information comes a great deal of BMD—bias, misinformation, and disinformation. As a patient, you may find yourself on your own as you scrounge the internet for information on your health, finding millions of hits that do more to scare and confuse you than inform you. We've seen this confusion most recently with the COVID pandemic, where we've been bombarded with conflicting information. "Where did it start, in the open market or the lab in Wuhan?" "Was it intentional germ warfare, an accident, or a natural mutation?" "It's just like the flu, no big deal!" "It will kill you if you get it!" "Masks don't work, masks make you sick, masks save your life." "What about Ivermectin?" "Are the vaccines safe? How many do we need? Will they make you infertile? Will they make you magnetic?" This "BMD" has resulted in too many illnesses, injuries and deaths, not just in the United States, but throughout the world.

There is bias, misinformation and disinformation in urology, as well. In writing this book, I want to be clear that I will declare my bias and try to be transparent about it. In those cases, I present alternative views and provide the data and reasoning that support my positions. There are many areas of medicine that are not black or white, with no single absolute right answer. Medicine is an art as much as a science, and as physicians we must draw conclusions and make decisions involving a number of differing factors. That's why shared decision making is so important—the more your physician knows about you and your unique needs, the more likely the decisions you make together will be the best decisions for you. By sharing my own biases in areas where I know there are differing views, the better equipped you'll be to draw your own conclusions.

But before you can draw any informed conclusions about your urological health, you need to know something about your own plumbing. So pour yourself a hot or cold drink, turn the page, and let me tell you how that drink is going down . . .

# CHAPTER 1

# Your Body's Plumbing

If you think of your central nervous system as your body's electrical system and your gastrointestinal system as your body's waste management system, then it makes sense to think of your genitourinary system as your body's plumbing system. Why think of something as complex as the human body in such simplified abstract terms? Because thinking of your body in this way makes it easier to understand. And because for all the wonders of the human body, it's basically a mechanical system of inter-related parts that function interdependently to keep you alive—until, of course, one or more of those parts breaks down. That's when you call someone like me, a urologist, to diagnose the problem and propose one or more ways to fix it.

Understanding your body's plumbing may help you to make decisions about your medical care. If you possess an appreciation of your anatomy and physiology, the decisions you make with your doctor will be more informed than the typical, "Oh, just do whatever you think is right Doc, and get it over with," response. We doctors appreciate a patient who understands how his body is put together and takes an active role in her treatment. So how is your genitourinary system put together? Let's start with the basic parts, sort of like figuring out what all these parts are to the Ikea product you just bought and have to put together.

There are eight basic parts we're going to talk about in this book: the adrenal glands, the kidneys, the ureter, the bladder, and the urethra. Whether you're having a problem urinating, suffer from kidney stones or a related cancer, one or more of these organs or parts will be affected. So let's take a look at where they are and what they do.

Remember that glass of water (or whiskey) I suggested you pour at the end of the Introduction. Well now's the time to drink it. Take a good long sip of your water, or a more modest sip of your whiskey, and feel it pass your lips, wet your tongue and glide down your throat until you can no longer feel it. Now that you can no longer feel it, what's it doing in the darkness of your inner body?

As that liquid flows down your throat, it already starts its work hydrating your mouth, esophagus, and stomach. As it does so, your brain receives signals that you are becoming hydrated. That's why after only a few sips of water, you might feel as if you've had enough—even if you really do need more. But if your brain didn't tell you you'd had enough early on, you'd keep drinking, potentially consuming too much by the time your brain was happy. It's going to take time for all the cells in your body to become hydrated by that drink, which is why your brain wants you to drink slowly—and steadily—throughout the day.

Your esophagus is a tube that connects your mouth to your stomach. As you fill your stomach with the fluid you are drinking, the fluid is transported to your small intestines, where it is absorbed and then enters your bloodstream.

Fluid absorption starts once the liquid reaches the small intestines (small intestines are about 20 feet long and stuffed inside of you like one of those collapsible hoses shoved inside a garbage bag at the end of the summer).The large intestines are wrapped around the small intestines like a frame. Fluid/water absorption continues in the large intestine and it's here in the that the cells in your body get the most benefit (or cost) from whatever it is that you're drinking, as the liquid reaches your bloodstream and hydrates your organs, tissues, muscles and cells.

Once your body has absorbed all the water it needs, it needs to get rid of what it doesn't need. There are four ways your body eliminates water: through your large intestines, in the form of feces; through your mouth, in the form of saliva; through your skin in the form of sweat; and through your kidneys in the form of urine. It's this last process we're concerned with here, as the water now in your bloodstream reaches your urinary tract.

The urinary tract starts in the abdomen in the space called the retroperitoneum. Retro means "behind," so the retroperitoneum refers to the space behind the peritoneum. The peritoneum is the abdominal space where your guts (stomach, small intestine, and parts of the large intestine), liver, and spleen reside. Also housed in the retroperitoneum are lymph channels running alongside your blood vessels and carrying lymph fluid, which is a byproduct of the filtration of blood returning to the heart. Situated along the course of the lymph channel are lymph glands. These lymph glands filter the lymph fluid. These lymph glands and channels become important if cancer invades the bladder, kidneys, uterus or ovaries, because if the cancer invades them, the cancer can spread to the pelvis and throughout the retroperitoneum. For this reason, certain cancer surgeries call for the removal of these glands and channels.

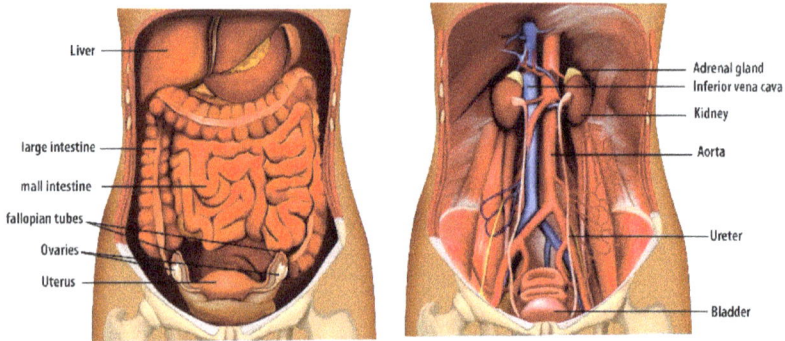

**Normal female anatomy of peritoneal (L) and retroperitoneal (R) cavity**

The urinary tract itself consists of the kidneys, ureters, bladder, and urethra. Your kidneys are two bean-shaped organs, each about the size of two fists pressed together. Your two largest blood vessels, the aorta and vena cava, supply blood to the kidneys through the renal arteries, and take blood back to the vena cava and eventually the heart via the renal veins. On top of your kidneys are your adrenal glands, which are shaped liked large fortune cookies. These glands produce three important hormones—steroids, adrenaline, and noradrenaline—which regulate your heartbeat, blood pressure, and serve other critical functions. Water reaches your kidneys through the bloodstream, just as it reaches other organs in your body. Without water reaching every organ, muscle and tissue, we'd be mummified inside. Unlike other organs in your body, the kidneys play a particularly important role in maintaining hydration and water balance throughout your body. Your kidneys also filter your blood and regulate vitamins, minerals, enzymes and hormones needed to stay alive, such as renin, an enzyme that regulates blood pressure and erythropoietin, a hormone that helps produce red blood cells. The kidneys also activate Vitamin D. No wonder you're in trouble if you have a problem with your kidneys! So how do they do all this?

Well, to simplify the process, once the water you've consumed is absorbed into your bloodstream, it reaches your kidneys via a series of arteries, which enter the kidneys into a vast network of microscopic blood vessels (arterioles). These tiny vessels are intwined with approximately two million tiny nephrons, which form a powerful network of detectors and filters. These nephrons identify anything the body needs, which is then reabsorbed by the nephron. Anything your body doesn't need, like urea (a byproduct of proteins), as well as any excess water your body doesn't need, is eliminated by the nephron. The combination of water and waste products that you don't need is urine.

Chemicals, salts (such as sodium and potassium), toxic waste, amino acids, vitamins, glucose, water, and other elements are regulated by the nephrons. Some of these substances, compounds, and electrolytes are filtered and excreted in the urine, while some are reabsorbed and put back into the bloodstream. Others are "regulated" so that just the right amount winds up back in the bloodstream. The nephrons add excess water to the things your body doesn't need to make urine. The more excess water you have in your body, the more hydrated you are, the more light-colored the urine will be. In contrast, the less hydrated you are, the more cloudy or dark your urine will be, given there is less water to dilute the waste products your kidneys are trying to eliminate.

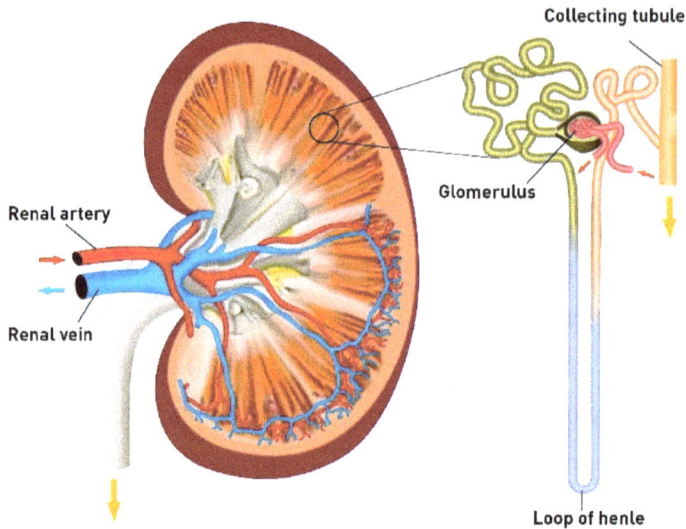

**Kidney (L) and glomerulus (R) anatomy**

That water and waste (now part of urine) travel through the ureters, which are foot long tubes about the diameter of a pencil that connect each kidney to the bladder. The inner lumen of each ureter is about 2 mm. (To give you some perspective, a common knitting needle and the tip of a new crayon are 2 mm, or 0.08 inches.)

Your bladder is a hollow muscle-walled organ that rests on your pelvic floor and temporarily stores your urine. It has three openings—the two openings where the ureters drain urine into the bladder, and the urethra, through which the urine leaves the bladder. The bladder is passively stretched until it reaches full capacity. When your bladder is full, it sends a message up the spinal cord and to the brain telling your brain that your bladder is full and you need to pee. When that happens, as soon as you sit on the toilet, your brain turns off the inhibitory fibers that travel down the spinal cord, the valves open, your bladder muscle contracts, and your pee is released, much to your relief.

A woman's urethra is two inches long, whereas a man's is ten to twelve inches long. The discrepancy between male and female urethras explains why women get more bladder infections than men. Bacteria that are normal inhabitants of the vaginal and anal areas have a much shorter distance to travel. The urethra transports the urine you eliminate from your bladder, by passing through the pelvic floor, ending at the vaginal opening.

## Conclusion

Of course, this whole description of your body's plumbing is an overly simplified thumbnail sketch of all that's going on inside but provides you with a basic understanding of the urological network that we urologists do our best to keep in good working order. By understanding how your body works, you are better able to make informed decisions about your healthcare. The better you understand your anatomy and how your body functions, the better you can assess potential risks, complications, and benefits of your treatment, including the medicines prescribed to you and any surgical options.

No matter what your urologic problem or issue may be, whether a kidney stone, blood in your urine, incontinence or a urinary infection, it helps to have a sense of how all your relevant body parts connect and function. In the chapters that follow, we'll look more closely at your particular concerns, where I provide more detail of your anatomy and how these various components of the urinary tract function—and what it means when one or more of these parts break down.

# CHAPTER 2

# I'm Peeing Blood!

Urologists deal with urine. We specialize in many other areas as well, but urine is our bread and butter so to speak. As you can imagine, we tell a lot of jokes about pee in the operating room and among friends and colleagues. From "Four out of five urologists smell their apple juice before they drink it," to "What did the urologist say to the patient who forgot to take his medicine? Urine trouble!" Well, if you're reading this chapter, you just might have urine trouble. If that's the case, rest at ease. There are many reasons you might be having urine trouble, most are easily treated, and if you do have a serious disorder, you're living in the best medical era of all time and there are many treatment options for even the most serious cases.

One of the more common reasons a patient is referred to a urologist is because they have blood in their urine, a condition known as "hematuria." For the patient, blood in the urine is quite frightening, but blood in the urine doesn't necessarily mean there's a serious problem. But it is important to find out why there is blood in the urine.

Although the urologist usually has a good idea why the patient was referred and what the primary care provider's (PCP's) concerns were, we like to have a good understanding of what the patient has experienced. For that reason, I usually start my visit with a conversation that goes something like this.

"Hi, Ms. So-and-So, I'm Dr. Lieberman. How are you today and how can I help you?"

The patient will usually greet me politely, but her face will be serious. "I have blood in my urine. I hope it's nothing serious."

Of course, they are usually pretty worried that it is indeed serious. My next question is aimed at learning more about just how serious it might be. In most cases, I'm able to alleviate their concerns, but they need to have it checked out. Blood in the urine isn't something to ignore.

"How do you know that you have blood in your urine?" I ask. The answer will give me important information. It's at this point that the conversation will diverge in several potential directions, which is why it's important to ask the question. Hematuria presents in a variety of ways, and how it presents gives us clues to what is going on.

The responses might be, "I saw some blood in the toilet a week ago, and then it went away. My urine is clear now, but I thought I should get it checked, just in case." Or, "I had burning and was peeing all the time, and then I saw some blood. My doctor gave me antibiotics and it cleared up, but she referred me to you. I think it's probably just from my UTI, but what do you think?"

In some cases, they didn't know they had blood in their urine until their PCP told them. "My doctor did a UA," they might say, referring to a urine analysis, "and told me I have microscopic blood, but I've never seen it." Or maybe it's more along the lines of, "I've had microscopic blood in my urine for years and they've given me all kinds of tests, IVP's (kidney x-rays with IV contrast or dye), CT scans, cystoscopies (a procedure done in the office under local anesthesia in which a flexible 5mm scope is passed through the urethra to the bladder), but they never find anything. That's why I've come to you. I need to know what's wrong." And in some cases, the patient has come straight to me after peeing a stream of urine as red as cabernet wine. Whatever the case, it's my job to determine where that blood is coming from and why it's there in the first place.

It's not uncommon for me to have already taken a look at their urine before I've even met the patient. We normally obtain a urine specimen before taking a history and doing a physical, and I would at times look at it prior to meeting the patient. It doesn't take much blood for urine to look pink, so with just one glance I can tell before it's even tested if there's blood. They taught us in medical school that if you couldn't read a newspaper through it (back in the days when newspapers were printed on paper, and not on computer screens!), then there was a significant amount of blood. Sometimes the specimen has clotted blood in it, which is an even greater concern. Whatever the state of the urine, if you can tell at a glance that the urine contains blood, it's called "gross hematuria."

Conversely, if the blood is not visible to the human eye and can only be observed through a microscope, we call it "microscopic hematuria." Whether you submit a urine specimen to the lab or we analyze it in the office, the specimen is first tested with a dipstick. The test strips measure not only blood, but also glucose, bilirubin, urobilinogen (two liver tests), ketones, leukocytes (white blood cells, which could indicate infection), nitrites (indicating the presence of bacteria), protein, and pH.

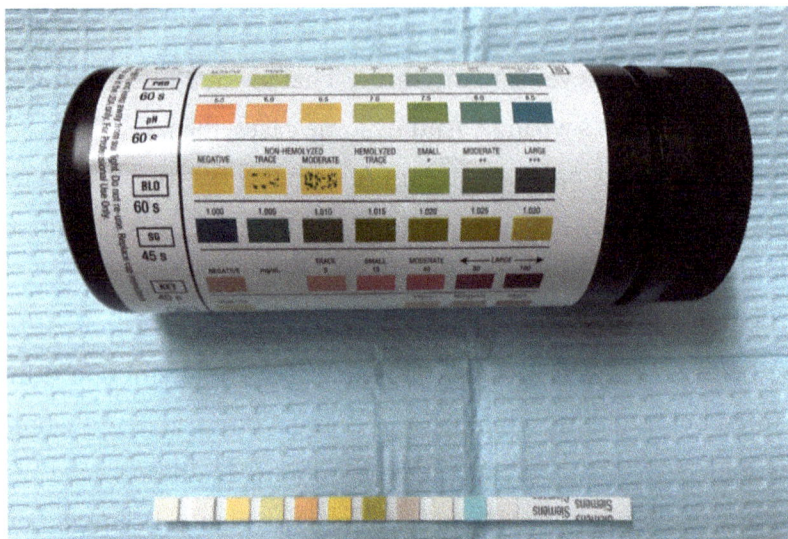

**The first part of a UA (urine analysis) is the dipstick. When the "blo" box turns green, it indicates the presence of blood.**

If the dipstick is positive for blood, the amount of blood is indicated by how dark green the dipstick box for blood becomes. The microscopic exam of the urine (done in most urologists' offices) will give us an accurate measure of the concentration of blood, or how many red blood cells are seen in each high-powered field. The specimen it then spun in a centrifuge, which concentrates the solid particles in the urine toward the bottom of the test tube. Those particles are put on a slide and either the lab tech or urologist (or both) examines it under a microscope, analyzing the number of red and white blood cells, crystals, and "casts" (think of a bunch of red or white cells stuck in a tube to form a "cast" of cells).

One thing that can complicate a UA (urine analysis) is how the urine specimen was obtained. Instructions are usually given to patients on how to collect the specimen, but sometimes the specimen is still contaminated by vaginal or external genitalia blood. We can usually tell when the specimen has been contaminated because there will be cells present that usually aren't present in urine. For women due to the proximity of the urethral opening to the vaginal opening, contamination is common due to improper collection, which is why it's so important to follow the instructions you're given for the urine collection.

Hematuria is sometimes associated with other symptoms—pain with urination, urinary frequency, urgency, frequently getting up at night to pee (nocturia), or pain anywhere along the course of the urinary tract from the kidney to the tip of the urethra. Sometimes hematuria will not be associated with any symptoms. This is called asymptomatic hematuria. Hematuria can also be chronic or acute. Why is any of this classification important? Why does it matter? If you have blood in your urine, shouldn't you see a urologist and have some tests to figure out why?

It matters because you don't want to have tests and X-rays that aren't necessary. Conversely, there are situations when you want to know what's causing the blood in the urine because there are certain conditions, particularly bladder and kidney cancer, that can be cured if diagnosed early, and possibly not cured if the diagnosis is delayed. Depending on what type of hematuria a person has, will determine the work up. Let's consider each type of hematuria starting with asymptomatic microscopic hematuria.

## Microscopic Traces of Blood

Asymptomatic microhematuria means that you cannot see blood in the urine with your naked eye, but blood has been found in the UA lab tests your physician ordered. If you've had no symptoms and couldn't see the blood, chances are you've been surprised by the lab results and you're worried that some silent killer might be lurking inside somewhere. Fortunately, that is usually not the case.

When I was in training, we were taught that any sign of microhematuria, no matter how negligible, necessitated a thorough and often uncomfortable workup that required an IVP and rigid cystoscopy (and often retrograde pyelograms - see glossary). It turns out, however, that a small amount of blood in the urine is quite common. Depending on how presence of blood is defined, the prevalence of microscopic blood in the urine is found in between 9% and 18% of patients. An estimated 25,000,000 Americans have blood in their urine. Blood in the urine is more common in older people and in smokers, but that doesn't necessarily mean there is anything wrong with them (although smoking is a definite risk factor for bladder cancer, which we discuss in Chapter 6).

In 2010, Ron Loo, M.D., one of my colleagues at Kaiser in Southern California, and I found that in over one million urinalyses done at Kaiser Southern California, almost one-third had evidence of hematuria, yet the evidence of bladder cancer for this same sample was less than one percent! We concluded that doing a urinalysis as a screening test for bladder or kidney cancer was a waste of time and resources—and was especially a disservice to our patients, because many of them were subjected to radiation from CT scans, and uncomfortable cystoscopies.

"Perhaps," you might be thinking, "but if there's even a slight chance of cancer, shouldn't follow-up tests be a good thing?" Not necessarily. Just think about it. I had been evaluating tens of thousands (or more) patients with asymptomatic microscopic hematuria for more than 35 years and never finding anything. But because I'd been trained that any indication of hematuria required a series of follow-up tests, these patients who had no other signs or symptoms of a disorder, and only trace amounts of microscopic blood in their urine, were subjected to tests with potential harmful radiation and dyes injected into them. They all had cystoscopy, which could be uncomfortable (particularly with the rigid cystoscopes we used in the 70s and 80s), and they had to take time off from work. Depending on their insurance some often had to pay hundreds, maybe thousands of dollars in copays and deductibles. Some of them, like airline pilots, whose routine flight physicals may have turned up microscopic blood in the urine, were unable to return to work until we cleared them. Yet even though I could predict with 99% accuracy that they were perfectly fine, they were subjected to these unnecessary tests, as well as all that worry.

For those who did have cancer, there were usually other signs and symptoms. For those patients, additional tests made sense. But for those who just have microscopic traces of blood in their urine with no other symptoms? My opinion was that we were subjecting these patients to unnecessary radiation and cystoscopy. Why then did we do it?

First, it was the standard of care at that time, and the one recommended by the American Urologic Association. Second, there was no financial incentive for either radiologists or urologists to rock the boat and say that a work-up for asymptomatic microhematuria was probably not necessary. Anyone who did rock that boat would be met with resistance from within the profession. Third, patients expected follow-up tests when blood was found and telling them they didn't need the tests, especially in light of the professional standards of the time would leave them feeling they were not getting adequate care. And finally, there was always the potential for litigation.

Some urologists would say (some still do say) that if they didn't evaluate a patient with asymptomatic microscopic hematuria and that patient was later diagnosed with cancer, then the physician who failed to do the CT scan and cystoscopy could be on the hook for a malpractice suit. So we erred on the side of caution and maintained a standard of care that subjected many patients to costly, uncomfortable, and sometimes risky tests that rarely revealed any serious problem. For years I was concerned that these tests were unnecessary. My fellow Kaiser urology chiefs and I launched a national study involving all Kaiser regions to determine how many patients with asymptomatic microhematuria had a serious problem. Our findings were more remarkable than I'd anticipated.

In the first year of the study, we collected data on 10,000 patients who had been referred by their PCP to a Kaiser urologist for "microscopic hematuria." We recorded six variables for all of these patients—age, sex, smoking history, amount of microscopic blood in the urine, presence of absence of symptoms, and whether or not the patient had a history of seeing blood in the urine with the naked eye (gross hematuria). All patients had cystoscopy and were subjected to imaging, usually a CT scan. We found that patients who had a history of gross hematuria were at the highest risk of having a malignancy. We were able to assign a risk score based on the variables of history of gross hematuria, sex (males are at greater risk), age (the older you are, the greater the risk), and smoking history. According to risk, we were able to divide the initial group of 10,000 into three groups based on risk factors (low, medium, and high). If a person had a history of gross hematuria within the past six months of being seen, they could not be in the low risk group.

There were 4,400 patients in the low risk group and only three malignancies were found among them. I went back and personally reviewed those three cases and it turns out that two of them did not have a malignancy after all, and one had a history of gross hematuria a year prior, but not in the past six months. Of the 10,000 in the initial group, 52 did have cancer, but all of them had a history of gross hematuria, and all were in the high risk group.

All this is to say, if your physician tells you that your lab work reveals blood in your urine and you've never noticed any indication of blood (that is, you've never had gross hematuria) and you have NO symptoms, it's highly unlikely that it's anything serious. On the other hand, CT scans involve a lot of radiation, which can cause cancer, so why have a test that you don't need?

I presented our findings at the annual American Urological Association meeting in 2013, and after the presentation, I sat down next to a urologist from Great Britain. He leaned over and said, "Very interesting talk, but we don't work up microhematuria in Europe, zero, none." Whether that is because they've known for some time that the workup for asymptomatic microhematuria is unnecessary, or that we have a privatized medical system that profits from expensive tests, it's hard to say.

As a result of our study, we developed a guideline at Kaiser for evaluating microscopic hematuria that has significantly reduced the number of unnecessary CT scans, cystoscopies, and days off work for unnecessary tests and appointments with a urologist. As a result of these new guidelines, we alleviated a lot of needless worry, not to mention the discomfort and financial strain of needless tests. But suppose the microscopic urine isn't the only thing going on? What if you have symptoms? If that's the case, you may indeed want further tests.

## Microscopic Blood in Urine with Other Symptoms

If you have microscopic blood in your urine along with other symptoms, we call it *symptomatic* microhematuria. What symptoms are we talking about? They can be specific to the urinary tract—pain or burning with urination, frequent urination, urgency, for example— or they may be more generalized "total body" symptoms such as fever, lethargy, malaise, or weakness. It's not uncommon for someone to go to their doctor for these generalized symptoms, have the doctor recommend a diagnostic workup, including blood and urine tests, and find the microscopic blood in the urine. In this case, a work-up is necessary.

Pain anywhere along the course of the urinary tract would trigger a urinary analysis (UA), assuming gynecological causes for the pain have been ruled out (such as blood from the uterus or cervix). There might be pain in the flank (kidneys, adrenals, ureters, and anything else in the retroperitoneum). Pain above the pubic bone might indicate a bladder infection. To learn more, it's important to consider your health history. Do you have a history of kidney stones? If so, there's a good chance that may explain the pain and hematuria. Maybe you have a history of UTI's? Whatever is going on, it's not something you can diagnose yourself, so you do need to see a doctor. Your physician will take your history and order a urinary analysis. Based on what's found in that analysis, if this is your first UTI, your doctor will treat your UTI and then recheck your urine for blood after the infection has resolve. If there is no UTI, a CT urogram will be done to see if the hematuria may be explained by kidney stones or something else. And you will need to see a urologist for cystoscopy in order to diagnosis the cause of your symptomatic microhematuria, if it's not due to a UTI.

Other symptoms might include frequent urination, burning with urination, urgency (feeling like you gotta go right now!), and getting up frequently at night to pee. These symptoms, when associated with microhematuria, might indicate bladder cancer, and should be evaluated with a CT scan and cystoscopy.

Whether or not you have other symptoms, what if the blood wasn't microscopic? If you notice visible blood in your urine, there still may not be a serious problem, but you definitely want to find out what's wrong.

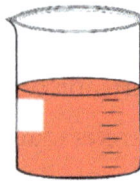

Gross hematuria means blood can be seen in the urine.

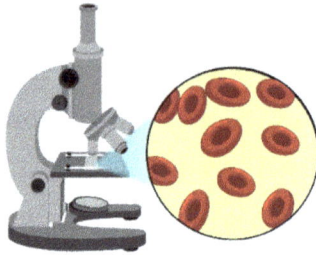

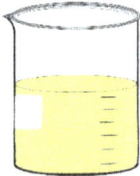

Microscopic hematuria means blood can be seen only with a microscope.

## Gross and microscopic hematuria

If you do see blood in your urine, you need to see a urologist. This condition is called gross hematuria. The blood may include visible clots, or can look like coffee grounds or cola. It may be pale pink, bright cherry red, dark burgundy, or bright orange. If the blood in your urine looks like coffee grounds, it's "old blood," meaning you are not actively bleeding, and the blood is likely coming from either the kidneys or bladder. If the blood in your urine is bright red, however, it means you are actively bleeding. Sometimes, particularly with bladder cancer, blood clots can be so voluminous that they will completely obstruct the bladder outlet and the patient can't pee at all. This is called clot retention and requires a urologist to irrigate the clots out. This requires a trip to the ER or urologist's office. In my experience, this is no fun for either the patient or the urologist.

Gross hematuria can occur at the beginning, middle, or end of the stream, or be present throughout the stream. If you notice blood in your urine, try to note when it happens, because that bit of history can be helpful in trying to determine where the blood is coming from. This may be a bit difficult for you because women sit down to pee and then see the blood in the toilet. If you aren't menstruating, you may assume that the blood is in the urine, but it may have come from the uterus, cervix, or vagina. Women are also more prone to urinary tract infections, which can be associated with gross hematuria.

If the blood appears in a steady stream, or begins clear and turns dark, then the problem could be further up in your genitourinary tract. Your urologist will want to check your kidneys and bladder with a CT and cystoscopy. While there is certainly cause for concern, the problem could be from an infection or stone, but it could also be something more serious like kidney or bladder cancer.

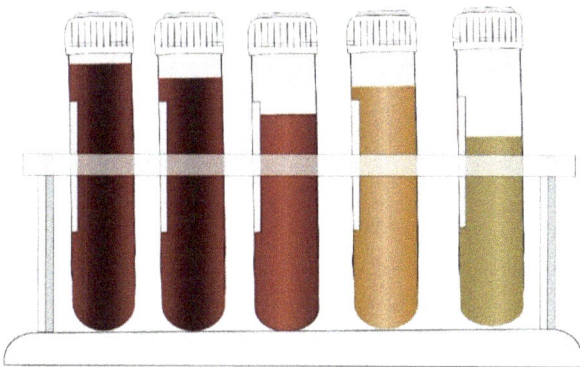

**Various degrees of gross hematuria**

As you can see, blood in the urine takes many forms. To keep it simple, if you are told "you have blood in your urine" you might be initially alarmed, but if you have no symptoms and have never seen blood in your urine, rest assured that you likely have nothing significantly wrong. However, if you *do* see blood in your urine, please seek professional medical help soon. If you have symptoms and your doctor says you have microscopic blood in your urine and recommends further evaluation, I'd advise that you do it, whether it's a renal ultrasound or CT urogram, and a visit to the urologist for a 15 minute procedure called cystoscopy.

A CT urogram is a CT scan that makes it possible to visualize the kidneys, ureters and bladder. For the procedure, a dye will be injected into your arm or hand, so that the radiologist can observe how it courses through and lights up the kidneys, then drains down the ureters and into the bladder. You may feel a rush of warmth from the dye but the procedure itself is painless, aside from the prick of the needle at the injection site.

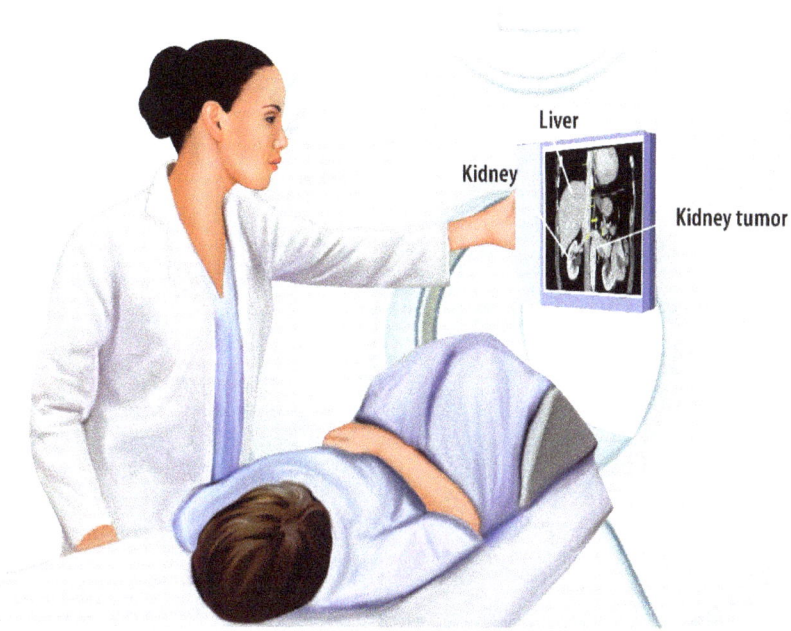

**CT scan of kidneys showing right kidney tumor and thrombus (clot) in renal vein**

Cystoscopy involves your urologist inserting a flexible 5 mm fiber optic scope through your urethra and into your bladder. Prior to the procedure, you'll be asked to empty your bladder. Your genitals will be prepped with a sterilizing solution (usually iodine based). A local anesthetic gel will be instilled into your urethra. You won't see the urologist for 10-15 minutes while the numbing agent does its thing. Once your urethra is numb, the urologist will insert the scope, which is attached to a camera. An image (of your urethra and bladder) is displayed on a screen, so you both can see what's up there. Then sterile water will flow through the scope into your bladder and fill your bladder to give your urologist a good view. You'll feel like you have to pee but try to relax and hold it.

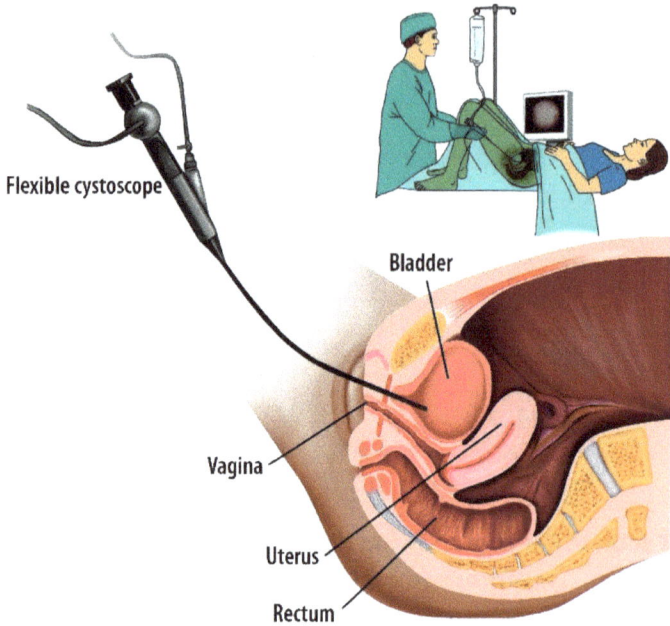

**Female Cystoscopy**

The procedure may sound awful, but you'll have to trust me on this one, it's not that bad. I've had four cystoscopies for gross blood in my urine due to stones in my prostate. It's mildly uncomfortable but not particularly painful. And it's a lot easier for women because the urethra is so much shorter than a male urethra.

## Conclusion

While you absolutely need to see a doctor whenever you see blood in your urine, don't panic. The cause could be from something benign. Blood in the urine means something is going on with the genitourinary tract, but that something might be a urinary tract infection (UTI), kidney or bladder stones (excruciating, but temporary), a sexually transmitted disease (STD's), or can even be caused by some medications (such as blood thinners or sulfa containing drugs). In other words, there might be a serious problem, but chances are, it's not, particularly if you have asymptomatic microscopic hematuria. If you have gross hematuria however, don't wait—the sooner you know why you have blood in your urine, the sooner you can get started on an early course of treatment if it is serious. In subsequent chapters I'll discuss these more serious concerns should it turn out that you have a tumor one of your kidneys, bladder, or elsewhere in your genitourinary tract. But for now, know that microscopic blood in the urine is common, and in most cases, not an indication of cancer, especially if there are no symptoms associated with it. If you can see it, it is a literal red flag giving you a shot at early detection.

# CHAPTER 3

# Incontinence and Overactive Bladder

One of the most common medical issues an adult woman may face in her lifetime is urinary dysfunction. Although not life-threatening, leaking urine, having to use the bathroom frequently, or not being able to control your bladder when you need to pee can have serious impacts on your daily living activities, your social life, your job, and your relationships.

This chapter will address the various forms of incontinence, sometimes associated with frequency and/or urgency. We'll also discuss frequency and urgency that can occur without loss of urine or with loss of urine. This is called an "overactive bladder" or OAB. Last, we'll look at an uncommon cause of urinary dysfunction that can occur in women called **interstitial cystitis**. Along the way we'll repeat a caveat—many of these symptoms can be caused by a disease process that affects the nervous system (multiple sclerosis and diabetes are two good examples).

The job of the bladder is to store urine, and then when full, empty completely. The bladder normally fills passively under low pressure. When it reaches capacity (about 400 ml or a little over 12 ounces in an adult female), a message is sent to the brain via peripheral nerves. The message travels up the spinal cord to the brain, alerting the brain that the bladder is full and needs to empty. The brain then looks for a place to pee, all the while inhibiting the contraction of the bladder until an appropriate place is found. The brain sends a message down the spinal cord telling the bladder to contract, while at the same time releasing the inhibition to contract. This is associated with an increase in bladder pressure. The brain also sends a message to the two valves that normally keep urine stored in the bladder telling them to open and let the bladder empty. When anything disrupts the message from bladder to brain and back down again to the bladder and valves, you get bladder storage problems. Storage problems also result from an anatomic abnormality in the bladder or valves.

When urine leaks, the condition is called **incontinence**. Urinating too often is a symptom we call **frequency**. Having the urge to go before the bladder has reached capacity is called **urgency**. Having to sit there a long time before anything happens is called **hesitancy** and is often seen with a slow stream and a feeling of not emptying completely. These symptoms can be seen in isolation or together. For example, you can have frequency, urgency, and be incontinent all at once. If you do have these symptoms, you are likely quite unhappy and could be helped by a urologist. Let's take the symptoms one at a time and discuss their causes and potential fixes. Even having one of these symptoms by itself can make for a miserable life, and possibly an expensive one if you are always having to wear Depends.

## Incontinence

There are three types of urinary incontinence in women—**stress incontinence**, which is when urine leaks when you cough, sneeze, or engage in any activity that causes an increase in intra-abdominal pressure; **urge incontinence** or getting the urge to go and not being able to hold it; and **overflow incontinence**. If you fill a glass of water to the top and keep filling it to the point that it overflows, that's overflow incontinence. Let's start with stress incontinence.

## Female Stress Urinary Incontinence

Women who have stress incontinence (leaking urine when you cough, sneeze, or anything that increases pressure in the bladder), have a normal functioning external sphincter. So why do some women leak when they laugh, cough or sneeze, and others don't? Imagine drawing a horizontal line across the pubic bone.

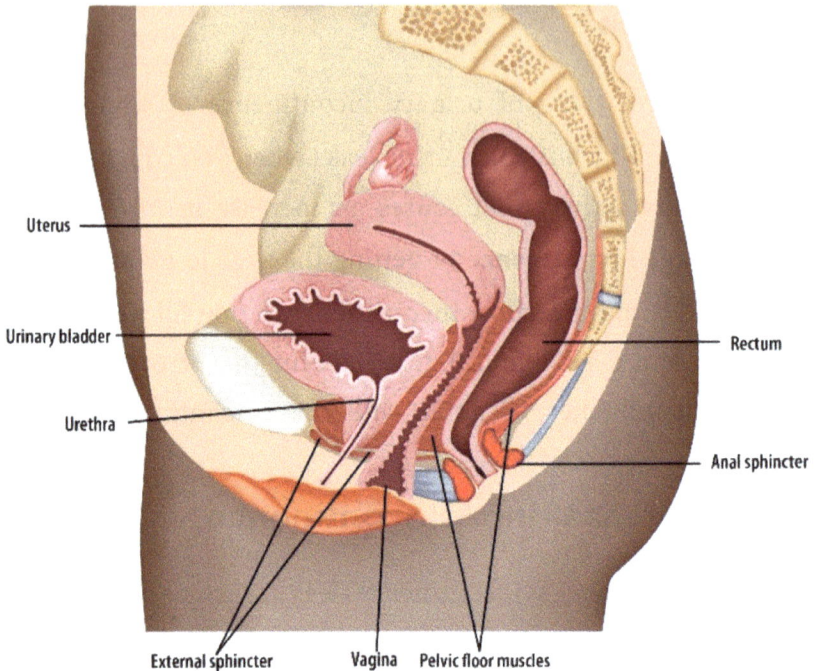

Uterus

Urinary bladder

Urethra

Rectum

Anal sphincter

External sphincter

Vagina

Pelvic floor muscles

## Normal female anatomy

All the structures and organs above that line are subjected to increased pressure in the abdomen and pelvis whenever you cough, sneeze, or laugh. Everything below that line receives no pressure when you cough, sneeze, or laugh. If the junction of the bladder and urethra (which is the same as the bladder neck and internal sphincter) and the external sphincter (which is the same as the pelvic floor) is above that line, you will not leak any urine when you cough, sneeze or laugh. But if the bladder neck (same as the internal sphincter) and external sphincter have dropped below that line due to a condition called "pelvic relaxation," when you cough there is increase pressure on the bladder (which is still above the line) but there is no pressure on both sphincters, so the pressure difference results in a leak.

The main reason for why this "bladder drop" has happened in the first place is because pregnancy and vaginal delivery of babies weakens the muscles of the pelvic floor and external sphincter. To fix a urine leak that happens with cough, sneeze, physical straining (really anything that increases intra-abdominal pressure) both sphincters (internal - bladder neck, and external - pelvic floor) need to be put back in their normal anatomical position, or above the magic line, or toward the head.

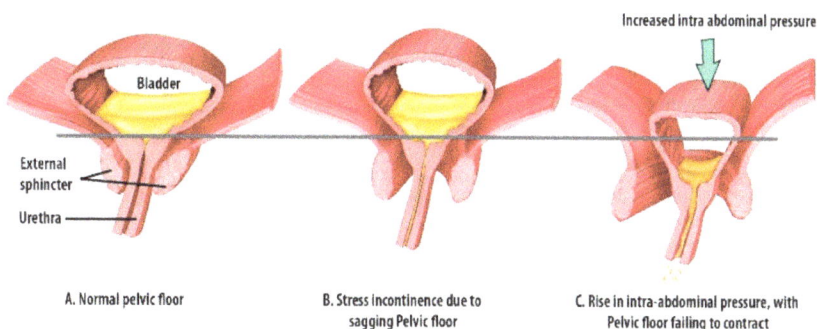

Increased intra abdominal pressure

Bladder

External sphincter

Urethra

A. Normal pelvic floor

B. Stress Incontinence due to sagging Pelvic floor

C. Rise in intra-abdominal pressure, with Pelvic floor failing to contract

Stress urinary incontinence occurs when the internal sphincter (junction of bladder neck and urethra) descends below the "magic line" (grey line) and is no longer subjected to intra-abdominal pressure

## Stress urinary incontinence

Another way to fix a urine leak is to inject a substance that will bulk up the junction of the bladder and the urethra (bladder neck). We'll talk about each of these methods, the attendant benefits, risks and drawbacks of each.

When you go to a urologist or uro-gynecologist seeking help for incontinence, what can you expect? Like all doctor visits, expect a complete history and a physical of your abdomen and pelvis. If you have neurological symptoms and there's a possibility that the bladder dysfunction and leakage could be due to a neurological problem (such as multiple sclerosis, spinal cord compression, or even diabetes), the doctor may also do a neurological exam. A urine analysis will be done to rule out an underlying infection and/or blood in the urine. S/he will probably see how well you empty your bladder with a "bladder scanner" which is a small ultrasound machine. If there is a small amount of "residual urine" (the amount of urine measured in your bladder by ultrasound or catheterization after you pee), then we've pretty much ruled out overflow incontinence. If there is a large residual, then overflow incontinence is a possibility, and we'll need to figure out why you aren't emptying your bladder.

Sometimes, especially if surgery is being considered to fix an incontinence problem, the urologist will do a test called a **cystometrogram**. A cystometrogram is done by placing a special catheter in the bladder. The bladder is then filled with either saline or dye. The special catheter measures pressure, and if there is fluoroscopic x-ray available, the doctor can simultaneously watch with intermittent x-ray images as the bladder fills. Normally the bladder will fill to capacity under low pressure. This is recorded on a graph. The doctor will ask you when you feel like you first need to pee. This volume at this point is recorded as the "first sensation to void." S/he will ask you when you feel the first urge to reach a toilet. This is called "urge." Then, when bladder capacity is reached and you feel like you can't hold it anymore and really have to go, the doctor may remove the catheter after noticing a spike in pressure. This is called the detrussor spike. At this point, if you aren't already leaking, s/he may ask you to cough or strain to document stress urinary incontinence.

At this point, a simple test called the Bonney test can be done. With approximately one cup of saline in the bladder, you will be asked to cough or strain while lying down in the lithotomy position (in stirrups like when you have a pap smear). The doctor will note if there is leakage. If there is s/he will note if the leakage occurs with the cough or strain, if it occurs shortly after, or both. If leak is present with cough, s/he will insert a finger or instrument into roof of the vagina alongside the urethra bladder junction. S/he will gently push up toward the ceiling to see if the leak with cough or sneeze can be stopped. It's important that the finger or instrument does not compress the urethra. The Bonney test simulates what the goal of present day urethral sling or suspension surgery tries to accomplish, that is, getting the sphincters above the magic line where they are subject to intra-abdominal pressure.

It's not uncommon for an element of urge incontinence to be present with stress incontinence. Sometimes the urge component can be treated with medication. For our purposes, I'd like to address the types of incontinence separately and discuss urge incontinence with the discussion of an overactive or neurogenic bladder.

Some women are not ready or interested in surgery. Their stress incontinence may be only occasional or very mild, or they may not be good candidates for surgery because of other medical problems. Instead of subjecting these patients to diapers or Attends, I'd sometimes recommend that they take two tampons and place them into the vagina. This accomplishes the same goal, that is, getting the sphincters above the magic line where they are subjected to the same increased intra-abdominal pressure that's exerted on the bladder itself with a cough or sneeze. You might think that the tampons block or obstruct the urethra. They don't. It's more of a repositioning phenomenon. If you do this, however, remember to remove the tampons after a few hours to prevent toxic shock syndrome.

Kegel exercises can strengthen the external sphincter muscle and even thicken the muscle. Kegels do the same thing to the external sphincter as doing curls in the gym does for your biceps. Kegels can sometimes fix mild cases of female stress urinary incontinence, but often more intervention is required. A referral to a physical therapist who specializes in pelvic floor strengthening exercises can help, as well.

There are two basic methods of fixing stress urinary incontinence—injecting bulking agents (such as bulkamid or coaptite), or a pubovaginal sling procedure.

Bulkamid is currently the most popular bulking agent. It's a procedure that can be done in the doctor's office under local anesthesia in about 15 minutes. Bulkamid is a polyacrylamide hydrogel (part of it is water) and is a popular agent used in plastic surgical procedures. It is biocompatible, nontoxic, and doesn't get reabsorbed into the body. The positive response rate has been reported to be greater than 65%, however in many cases the durable response doesn't last beyond two years. While the temporary benefit might make the procedure less attractive for most women, for elderly patients or women with multiple medical problems who may not tolerate a general anesthetic, Bulkamid may be a valuable thing for these patients to consider.

If Bulkamid isn't the right choice, the other option is surgery, specifically a pubovaginal sling procedure. A sling essentially repositions the sphincters (internal and external) to a more physiologic and more functional anatomic place. Let's take a closer look at what this procedure entails.

## Surgery to Correct Stress Urinary Incontinence

The most common and popular surgery to correct incontinence is called a mid-urethral sling. The goal of this procedure is to elevate the junction of the bladder and urethra back behind the pubis. There are several types of material the surgeon can choose from to use as the sling, including synthetic mesh, human cadaver tissue, or your own tissue (called autologous fascia which is the tough tissue that envelops your muscles—this tissue is harvested from your own abdominal wall muscle called the rectus). The sling can be anywhere from 5-6 cm (about 2.3 inches) up to 10 cm long and about 1 cm wide (about the size of your index finger).

The material your urologist uses for the sling depends on patient factors and surgeon preference and experience. This is true for the three placement procedures of slings (TVT, TVO, and single incision mini-sling). With all three procedures, small incisions are made in the roof or ceiling of the vagina and two small incisions are made either above the pubic bone or alongside the labia. Needles are passed through these incisions and sutures attached to each end of the sling are passed through the eye of the needles. The sling is then placed under the middle of the urethra in the shape of a hammock. With the bladder full and gentle pressure applied to the lower abdomen, the sutures are pulled up with just enough tension to stop any leak.

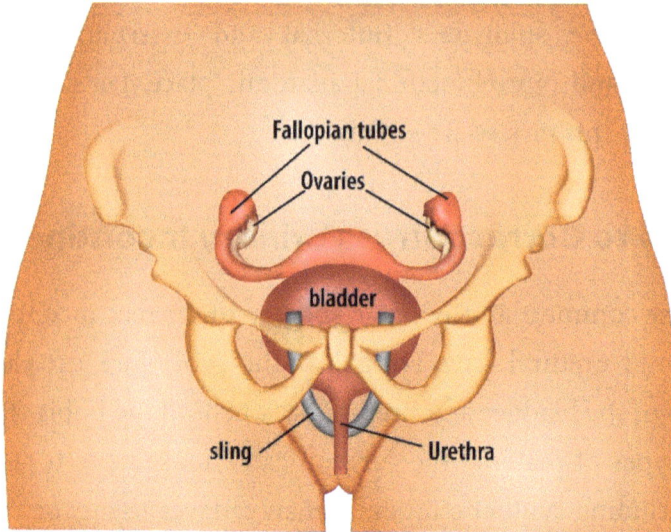

Pubo-vaginal sling positions the internal sphincter (junction of bladder and urethra) above the "magic line" to keep you dry when you cough, sneeze, or laugh

## Pubo-vaginal sling

Mid-urethral sling surgery has been around for over 20 years and due to advances in technology and techniques, there are fewer complications. While complications still happen, they are uncommon, and include urinary retention (sutures pulled up too tight or a lot of swelling around the urethra), wound infection, erosion of the sling into the urethra, and injury to the bladder or ureters during needle placement. Other rare complications include bleeding, infection of the sling, or new voiding symptoms like urgency. UTIs can also occur after a sling, particularly if bladder emptying is impaired. Very rarely a segment of bowel can be perforated.

Sometimes the muscles of the pelvic floor supporting the vagina, uterus, and cervix, have become so stretched and weakened by vaginal deliveries and perhaps obesity, "prolapse" will occur and accompany stress incontinence. When this weakness involves the roof of the vagina, the bladder, which is above the vagina, will prolapse into the vaginal vault. This is called a cystocele. If this is significant enough, during sling placement the surgeon will tighten the top of the vaginal wall with a procedure called an anterior repair ("repairing the roof" so to speak). If it's the floor, the rectum, which is underneath the vagina, will prolapse into the vault. This is called a rectocele, and to fix it a "posterior repair" ("repairing the floor") is done. At the back or end of the vagina is the cervix which is part of the uterus. When the uterus/cervix comes down into the vagina, the gynecologist may recommend a suspension procedure that fixes the uterus to the sacrum. This is called a culposuspension and can be done laparoscopically or daVinci robot assisted laparoscopically. In these instances, the surgery is more involved so there are more potential complications. That's why it's important to choose a surgeon who is trained and experienced. Pelvic organ prolapse, whether it involves one organ or all three, is frequently associated with one or numerous forms of voiding dysfunction—stress and/or urge incontinence, overactive bladder, or incomplete emptying. Fortunately, surgical correction often improves or cures these problems.

## Urge Incontinence and Overactive Bladder

I'm going to talk about these two conditions together, because although they are not the same, they are closely related and frequently occur together.

If you have the sudden frequent urge to pee, even though you just went 30-60 minutes ago and your bladder couldn't be nearly full already, you may be suffering from an overactive bladder. If you have a sudden urge to pee, can't hold it and wet yourself, you have urge incontinence.

Overactive bladder (OAB) is defined as a frequent strong urge to urinate. This urge can occur during active daytime hours and sometimes during the night too. These symptoms are not life threatening, but they can be a real bother and very disruptive in many areas of your life. If this is you, you know what I'm talking about. Some of my most depressed and desperate patients were referred for overactive bladder. Having to run to the toilet frequently can disrupt your sleep, leaving you exhausted. It can interfere with your work and daily activities, and lead to depression and anxiety.

Ninety-five percent of people with overactive bladder are women (if you don't count men who have similar overactive bladder symptoms due to prostate enlargement). Since overactive bladder is more common but certainly not limited to old people, OAB can cause falls and broken bones as women hurry to the bathroom so they don't wet themselves.

I realize it can be an embarrassing thing to discuss with your doctor, but please don't hesitate to get help. There are many things we can offer to turn your life around. You may think it's part of natural aging and there's nothing we can do about it. This is just not the case. In fact, most overactive bladder symptoms can be managed by your PCP without the involvement or need for a urologist. What's more, a majority of OAB patients do not need further testing or procedures other than those done routinely by a PCP. A good history, physical (including neurological) exam, and a urine analysis, are enough to let your PCP know whether or not s/he should refer you to a urologist.

The causes of overactive bladder symptoms and urge incontinence are frequently never discovered. Let's look at why the bladder is behaving badly in some cases. The reasons are threefold:

1.  There is something in the bladder (like an infection, stone, or foreign body-something in there that shouldn't be) that's irritating the bladder and stimulating the bladder muscle to contract.

2.  The nerves going from the bladder to the brain and then spinal cord are oversensitive and not working properly by sending an incorrect message to the brain telling it that the bladder is full and it's time to go (again). The reverse could also be present, that is, bad information coming from the brain via the spinal cord and peripheral nerves telling the bladder to go and go now.

3.  The bladder muscle itself is hyperactive and spasms at inappropriate and inconvenient times. Again, in most cases we never find a specific cause, however, it's remains important to rule out potential causes.

Why? Because sometimes the cause (infection or UTI for instance) can be easily diagnosed and treated. Also, OAB and/or urge incontinence are sometimes the first sign of a neurologic disease. Common examples would be Parkinson's Disease or Multiple Sclerosis. Many patients who are known to have a neurologic condition will frequently have voiding difficulty, including OAB and urge incontinence. A stroke would be another example of how a neurologic condition can cause bladder dysfunction. Diabetes affects the peripheral nerves (the nerves going to and from the bladder to the spinal cord, and vice versa), which can result in voiding dysfunction like OAB and urge incontinence. Patients who have spinal cord injuries may suffer from voiding dysfunction. When the voiding dysfunction is related to a neurological condition, the bladder dysfunction is called "neurogenic bladder."

How is the diagnosis made? Your doctor will take a history and will pay close attention to any neurologic symptoms or history of neurologic problems you may have. S/he will also review your medications, because medications can cause OAB symptoms and urge incontinence. On physical exam s/he will look for signs of vaginal prolapse or atrophy and test your nervous system with a neurological exam. S/he will do a UA to rule out an infection and check to see how well you empty your bladder with an ultrasound or catheter (also known as "post void residual). If you are ultimately referred to a urologist, s/he will repeat those things. S/he may also look in your bladder and recommend a CMG, which stands for cystometrogram.

Before you get to a urologist however, your PCP can treat your overactive bladder, provided your urine is free of blood and infection, and your neurological history and physical are negative. The keys to treatment are behavioral/physical therapy in the form of Kegel's exercises (with or without vaginal weights), biofeedback, and drugs.

There are a variety of drugs that help patients with OAB.

- Tolterodine (Detrol)
- Oxybutynin, which can be taken as a pill (Ditropan XL) or used as a skin patch (Oxytrol) or gel (Gelnique)
- Trospium
- Solifenacin (Vesicare)
- Fesoterodine (Toviaz)
- Mirabegron (Myrbetriq)

All of them, with the exception of Mirabegron, are a variety of anti-cholinergic drugs. The compounds vary slightly so the effectiveness of each and the side effects will also vary. Anti-cholinergics work by blocking a chemical (acetyl choline) that is released by nerves where the nerves terminate in the bladder muscle. If the chemical (acetyl choline) is a key, and the bladder muscle is a lock, inserting the key into the lock causes the bladder muscle to contract. The drugs used to treat OAB block the key from entering the lock, and results in bladder muscle relaxation and fewer contractions.

Mirabegron works the same way but is specific for a different chemical (a so called alpha agonist), but it also causes bladder muscle relaxation. There are cholinergic receptors throughout the body. Since the drugs are not specific to the bladder muscle, they will cause side effects. The main side effects are dry mouth, dry eyes, and constipation. The drugs can also have a bad effect on your eyes if you have a certain type of glaucoma.

These drugs for OAB are usually taken by mouth and are metabolized by the liver. They also can be delivered to the body by way of a skin patch. The difference is that the medicine in the pills taken by mouth have to go through the liver. The medication delivered by the skin patch goes right to the bladder. I found in practice that the skin patch anticholinergics worked as well or better than the oral preparations, but with the added benefit of fewer side effects.

One word of caution about the chronic use of anti-cholinergic medication in middle age and older adults. Along with several other type drugs (such as anti-depressants, drugs used to treat Parkinson's Disease, and seizure medication, chronic anti-cholinergic use (longer than 2-3 months) has been associated with an increased incidence of dementia. If you are going to take them, take them only for the short term, or a few months, not years. Long term use of tropsium and mirabegron seem not to be associated with dementia.

When should you see a urologist? Once your PCP has determined that your OAB symptoms are not explained by an infection, that you have no neurological symptoms or signs on physical exam, and that you have no blood in your urine, your PCP may want to check you for atrophic vaginitis due to post-menopausal lack of estrogen and try topical estrogens to help your OAB symptoms. If these measures aren't helping, and you haven't responded to behavioral therapy or drugs, it's appropriate for you to see a urologist.

The urologist will repeat much of what the PCP has already done, looking for clues to determine what is causing your symptoms. In addition, s/he may want to look in your bladder (cystoscopy) and check the pressures and muscle activity of your bladder with a cystometrogram (CMG). S/he may want to try different medications or more intensive behavioral therapy.

If all else fails and you are still having symptoms that aren't explained by a definite cause, there is still hope. Botox, when injected into the bladder muscle, will relax the bladder muscle and lasts for several (if not more) months. A urologist needs to do these injections (as many as 50-75) through a scope, under vision, and usually under anesthesia.

If the sacral nerves are stimulated, this can also produce relief. This procedure is done by placing a temporary wire adjacent to the sacral nerve through the back part of the pelvis under x-ray guidance. The patient is given a box that's attached to the wire. When the nerve is stimulated it causes the bladder muscle to relax. If it works, a permanent wire is implanted.

Another novel treatment of OAB also involves stimulation of a nerve, only in this case the nerve that's stimulated is just above the ankle and does not innervate the bladder muscle. This is called PTNS which stands for posterior tibial nerve stimulation.

PTNS is highly effective therapy for OAB. It is more effective than drugs with fewer side effects. Over 80% of patients on medications for OAB will be able to discontinue medication within the first six months of treatment.

The reason PTNS works is based on the theory of "neuromodulation." Neuromodulation is the stimulation of nerves to affect secretion of certain chemicals or neurotransmitters and is used in a variety of specialties for pain relief and treatment of a variety of disorders including seizures, heart, and bowel problems. Acupuncture may be a form of neuromodulation.

Urge incontinence is an overactive bladder that is stronger than the sphincters that keep the urine in, thus a leak on the way to the bathroom because the urge can't be suppressed. Loss of urine occurs because the bladder contracts or spasms at the wrong time. Urge incontinence can occur no matter how much urine is in the bladder. Most of the time a specific cause cannot be found. However, potentially serious causes still need to be ruled out, such as a bladder stone, foreign body, bladder cancer, infections, nerve, spinal cord, or even brain problems (stroke or Parkinson's). One last point about OAB. The future of treatment for OAB is promising. There are currently stage III prospective randomized clinical trials underway using gene therapy injected into the bladder that affects muscle relaxation. Hopefully, by the time you read this chapter, if you are suffering from OAB, this promising new therapy will be available to you.

## Interstitial Cystitis

No discussion of bladder voiding problems would be complete without discussing interstitial cystitis. You may already have been diagnosed with IC. If so, you may be in search of more information and help regarding this frustrating condition. Or you may have frequency, urgency, and a painful bladder and have not yet been diagnosed with IC, but you are not improving with conservative treatments and/or the medications recommended by your doctor.

IC is also known as "the painful bladder syndrome" and frequently is accompanied by frequency, urgency, incontinence, and numerous trips to the bathroom at night. The diagnosis is often made by a characteristic appearance of the bladder during cystoscopy. When the bladder is filled, stretched and distended, the bladder lining takes on an appearance of significant inflammation—the lining is very red and can crack and bleed. Sometimes we'll see ulceration of the bladder lining (called 'Hunner's ulcer'). A bladder biopsy is necessary to confirm the diagnosis. Under the microscope there is evidence of severe inflammation that involves all three layers of the bladder—lining or mucosa; middle layers or smooth muscle; outer layer or serosa. This aggressive approach to diagnosing IC is not practiced by all urologists, however. Some urologists will prefer to make the diagnosis based on symptoms only. However, it's been my experience that these same symptoms can be confused with carcinoma (cancer) in-situ of the bladder, and we don't want to miss this or delay this diagnosis, which is why I preferred to do a biopsy.

IC is an illness that particularly benefits from a shared decision approach. IC is a chronic condition, and your symptoms may be significant, dramatically affecting the quality of your life. Since UTI symptoms are similar, negative urine cultures are necessary. Symptoms must be present for at least six weeks prior to entertaining the diagnosis of IC. During the history and physical exam, your doctor will rule out a potential neurologic condition which could account for the symptoms. Also, a bladder ultrasound to check residual urine and rule out urinary retention will likely be done. Your urologist may recommend cystoscopy, which is a five minute outpatient procedure. The procedure requires filling the bladder under local anesthesia which can be painful for IC patients, so some urologists will forego cystoscopy in the office and advise you to have the procedure done under anesthesia. A bladder biopsy to confirm the diagnosis can be done at the same time.

There are five levels of treatments for IC, ranging from simple behavioral methods, all the way to removal of the bladder in severe cases. Shared decision making should be directed toward improving your symptoms and quality of life, while limiting side effects of treatments. Many therapies have been tried for IC and no one treatment is a magic bullet, so expect that you'll need a combination of treatments. Finally, you should also be aware of several therapies that have been employed in the past that have been shown to have no benefit yet have significant side effects.

Let's start with the simplest treatments. Like incontinence, there are behavioral modification techniques and physical therapy done by a trained and skilled physical therapist that can help. However, unlike incontinence, Kegel's exercises or pelvic floor exercises don't help, and in fact can make IC symptoms worse.

Oral drugs (the list includes pyridium, tricyclic antidepressants like Elavil, cimetidine, hydroxazine, Elmiron, and Cyclosporin A) can help. The most common oral drug for IC is amitryptiline (Elavil). Elavil is a tricyclic anti-depressant but in controlled clinical trials, IC patients experience benefit. The same can be said for Elmiron, though there are potential significant complications associated with this drug that can affect vision (the drug affects the macula of the retina). Nevertheless, some patients respond to Elmiron, though they need to be followed by an ophthalmologist for retinal changes that may require discontinuation of the drug. Cyclosporin A has significant potential side effects, however, so it is usually reserved as a last ditch oral agent.

Added to oral drugs are medications that can be placed into the bladder. We use a "cocktail" of drugs instilled into the bladder weekly for six to eight weeks. Our "cocktail" contains DMSO, heparin, and lidocaine (a local anesthetic).

If medications don't work, we move on to general anesthesia with slow flow and low pressure distension of the bladder. One of the risks of doing this procedure is that the bladder could rupture. And there's no guarantee it will work. Some patients respond with significant improvement of symptoms, others don't. As we discussed in the section on overactive bladder, some IC patients will respond to injections of botulism toxin (Botox) into the bladder, or neuromodulation with posterior tibial nerve stimulation, or permanent sacral nerve stimulation.

Severe IC can result in a very small fibrotic bladder in which pliable muscle tissue is replaced by scar tissue. This may happen even after multiple types of treatment, and when it does, surgery may be necessary. There are a variety of procedures to increase bladder capacity using segments of intestine attached to the bladder. With end-stage disease it's sometimes necessary to remove the bladder entirely and divert the urine with a loop of intestine that empties into a bag, or a "new bladder" called a "neobladder" which is a bladder created out of intestine. You can read more on this type of surgery in the chapter on bladder cancer.

There are several treatments that have been tried in the past that don't work and can cause harm. These treatments should be avoided. If your urologist is recommending any of these, it's time for a second opinion. They include long-term antibiotics, BCG (a bacteria used for treatment of bladder cancer) instilled in the bladder, high-pressure bladder distention under anesthesia (which can rupture the bladder rupture and has inconsistent benefits), and long-term oral steroids. IC can be a chronic and difficult life altering problem to deal with. It's important to be able to communicate your goals and preferences with your doctor, and it's important for s/he to communicate the various options for treatments. Multiple treatments may be necessary and they all have attendant risks and benefits. Hopefully you will find the combination that will get you better.

## Urinary Retention

Finally, one other problem that is less common in women than in men is urinary retention. A female bladder can become obstructed due to severe prolapse, severe urethral narrowing (stricture or stenosis of the urethral opening), certain drugs, or a neurogenic bladder.    If the bladder becomes over-distended the muscle can be severely stretched. The bladder becomes flabby and may not be able to generate any pressure at all. This becomes important in cases of severe obstruction that results in the total inability to empty and is called "urinary retention." Bladder volumes normally range of 400 - 600 cc in women. In cases of retention, I've seen bladder volumes as high as 1-3 liters (one liter is about a quart). Urinary retention results in the last type of incontinence called "overflow incontinence." Initially an over distended and flaccid bladder needs to be emptied completely and allowed to remain empty using a catheter so that it can heal. The bladder muscle may never recover, and in this case bladder emptying is accomplished by intermittent catheterization 4-6 times a day.

## Conclusion

Wet pants and frequent trips to the bathroom are no fun. Add to these embarrassing and inconvenient symptoms a painful bladder in the case of interstitial cystitis, it's no wonder that these problems can significantly affect a woman's quality of life. Urologist and Uro-gynecologists are trained to diagnose and treat these conditions. I know that it can be embarrassing, but good help is available to help you overcome these problems. Sometimes, however, the problems you face aren't about incontinence at all, but about painful urination. If you've ever had a urinary tract infection, you'll want to read the next chapter.

# CHAPTER 4

# Urinary Tract Infections

An infection is caused by a bug. That bug can be a bacteria, a virus, fungus, or other rare germs. Infections cause the body to mount an inflammatory response in an attempt to rid the body of the bug. However, you can have inflammation without an infection, that is, sometimes we can't identify an organism or bug that's producing the inflammation.

A urologist will be able to tell the difference by doing urine analyses and cultures. How can you tell whether your urinary problem rises to the level of seeing a doctor or urologist? As we've discussed in Chapter 2, anytime you see blood in your urine, you need to see a urologist. Similarly, anytime you have pain when you pee, you need to see a doctor. But first, let's take a closer look at urinary tract infections (UTI), so that you have a better idea of why we want you to seek treatment as soon as possible.

The infection can be anywhere along the genitourinary tract, including the kidneys, bladder, ureters, and urethra. An infection in the bladder or urethra is considered a lower tract infection, while an infection in the kidneys is an upper tract infection. Lower tract infections are caused by bacteria that enter the urethra then migrate into the bladder. Though UTI's are rare in men, they're common in women given the shorter urethra. When a UTI does occur, it can become complicated and reach the kidneys, so they're nothing to mess around with. Most cases UTI's can be treated with antibiotics, and can be well managed and resolved by a primary care provider (PCP).

About 60% of women will have a UTI at some point in their life. The unpleasant symptoms of a UTI can include abdominal pain, burning when urinating, fever, cloudy or bloody urine, increased urgency, urgency without being able to pee, and smelly urine. If you have any of these symptoms, you need to see a doctor.

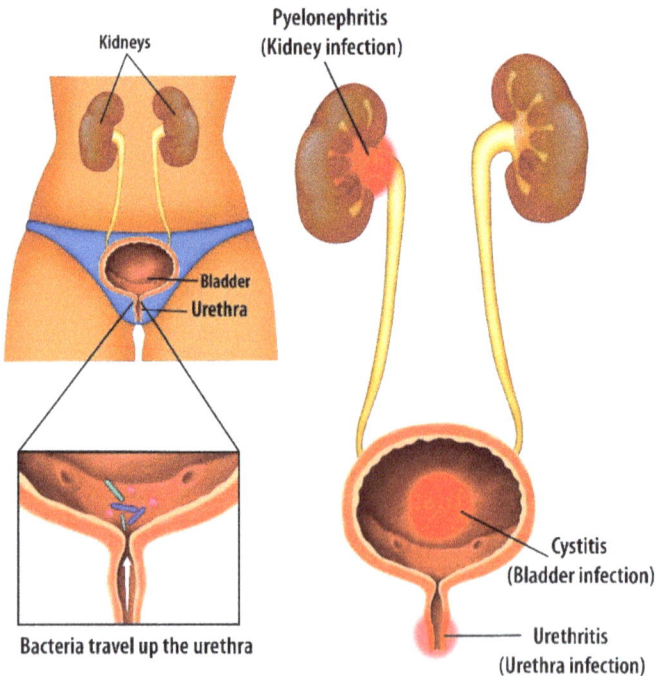

**Urinary Tract Infections**

One of the first steps your doctor will take is to determine what type of infection you have. There are many different kinds of UTIs, ranging from simple bladder infections to serious kidney infections or a kidney abscess. Some UTIs can become quite serious if the bacteria enter the bloodstream, in which case a condition called sepsis. Septic shock can result from a UTI, which is potentially deadly. For this reason, early diagnosis and treatment is imperative.

To assess the infection, your doctor will have you obtain a midstream clean catch urine specimen and either do a urine dipstick and microscopic exam in his/her office or send the specimen to a lab. A clean catch midstream sample means that after you clean around your urethra, you begin peeing into the toilet to clear the urethra, then in the middle of the stream you collect urine into the specimen container (more on this in a few paragraphs). Your doctor will also examine your genitals as well as palpate your abdominal area to feel for any lumps or tenderness.

If your infection is limited to the lower tract, it is often easily treated, but you want to catch it early so that it does not spread to the kidneys, in which case treatment can be more difficult. Given all these variables, let's consider the different types of urinary tract infections and how you can treat them.

## Cystitis

When bacteria get into the bladder they set up camp and cause an immune response. We call that cystitis, commonly referred to as a bladder infection. Cystitis is much more common in women than in men due to the shorter urethra (which is about 1.5 inches in women, and 7 to 8 inches in men). Because bacteria normally live in and around the vagina and anus, the bacteria can enter the bladder through the urethra. Bacteria also gain access to women's bladders during sex, which is another reason cystitis is more common in sexually active women. Cystitis can also be caused by a number of other factors – catheters, sexually transmitted diseases, difficulty emptying the bladder (stagnant urine or large post-void residual), diabetes, and poor hygiene.

When ascending bacteria get into the urethra they can cause an infection in the urethra or urethritis. Most of these infections are from sexually transmitted diseases and are due to chlamydia or gonococcal bacteria (gonorrhea), or a bug called *ureaplasma ureolyticum*. Most urethral infections are caused by STDs and can be treated by PCPs with antibiotics, and don't require the services of a urologist, unless they recur.

If you picked up a UTI from a sexually transmitted disease, the symptoms are typically limited to pain in the urethra and a discharge. One of the late complications that occurs after an infection in the urethra is that scar tissue, called a urethral stricture, can develop after urethritis. The narrowing in the urethra can be quite significant and appear like a pinpoint opening, whereas normally the inner diameter of the urethra is equivalent to a straw. A stricture that occurs after a bout of urethritis will usually result in one or more urinary symptoms: a slow trickling stream, difficulty starting a stream, frequent urination, getting the urge to go and feeling like you can't hold it, or feeling like you can't empty your bladder.

One cause of cystitis is an anatomic anomaly called a bladder diverticulum. This diverticulum can either be hereditary, or develop, and is a small, or not so small, sac or pouch in the bladder where urine pools and doesn't empty, again, allowing bacteria to grow. I've seen bladder diverticula that are twice the size of the actual bladder and hold up to a liter of stagnant urine—it's not hard to imagine how the bacteria that can take up residence in such a situation. A diverticulum can also occur in the urethra and is a potential explanation for recurrent UTIs in women. Last, other rare bugs can also cause urinary infections in women who have compromised immune systems.

Also, another cause of cystitis is a bladder stone(s). Bladder stones can be solitary or multiple and can range in size from a BB to as large as a tennis ball. Infections can also be caused by foreign bodies in the bladder. Usually these are pieces of previously placed urinary catheters or stents that have broken off and have not passed.

## Pyelonephritis

A bacterial infection can reach the kidney or kidneys one of two ways, either by ascending from the bladder to the kidney through the ureter (the tube that connects the kidney to the bladder), or via the bloodstream. A kidney infection is called pyelonephritis. Pyelonephritis can be serious. It is characterized by flank pain (pain in the kidney), and sometimes fever, nausea, and vomiting. So how do you get a kidney infection? It gets back to the possible causes of all UTIs—bacteria entering the bladder, stagnant urine, stones, or foreign bodies.

A kidney infection can also be associated with obstruction of the ureter anywhere along the one foot length of ureter from kidney to bladder, which in turn causes stagnant urine. The obstruction can be due to a stone, an acquired or congenital abnormality, or what we call an extrinsic cause. That means there is something outside the ureters that is causing the blockage. There are a variety of things that can cause this blockage ranging from benign enlargement of lymph nodes, to scarring from prior radiation therapy of the pelvis, to cancer. Other causes can include an infection from elsewhere in the body entering the bloodstream and reaching the kidneys.

Pyelonephritis needn't be serious, if caught early, provided there are no anatomic problems. It can usually be treated with a course of antibiotics and will clear up in one to two weeks, *provided the cause of the infection has been addressed.* If not diagnosed and treated early, however, the infection can cause permanent damage to your kidneys and cause scarring or even an abscess. What's more, if the bacteria enter your bloodstream, you may develop sepsis which, as I've stated earlier, can cause shock and even be fatal. Because infections can cause scarring to the kidneys, if left untreated or if the treatment is delayed or incomplete, the infection could lead to high blood pressure, chronic kidney disease and renal failure. For all these reasons, if you have flank pain and a urine analysis showing an infection (whether or not you have fever, nausea, and vomiting), *it's important to have an ultrasound of your kidneys.* The sooner an anatomic problem like an obstruction is diagnosed, the sooner you can have the obstruction relieved, and hopefully you'll avoid all the horrible things discussed above.

Pyelonephritis can also be caused by stones in one of two ways. Stones made of magnesium, ammonium, and phosphate produce what is called "infectious or struvite stone," that has a specific bacteria in it (*e. coli, pseudomonas,* or *proteus*). The only way to clear up the infection is to get rid of the stone. The other cause of pyelonephritis is an obstruction of urine drainage or a blockage anywhere along the drainage system from the junction of the renal pelvis and ureter, to the end of the urethra. When a blockage of urine drainage results in stagnant urine, an infection can occur. Finally, just as in the bladder and urethra, diverticula can also occur in the kidney and become infected.

## Bacteriuria

It's also possible to have bacteria in the urine and not have a UTI. This condition is called bacteriuria. Bacteria are in the bladder and urine but do not cause an infection or inflammation. Instead, they are passed into the toilet with urination or by emptying the bladder through a catheter. The condition of bacteriuria without a flagrant UTI is seen in some people with chronic indwelling catheters or double J stents. The urine is colonized by bacteria but you may not have any symptoms. If this is the case, it's not a good idea to treat the bacteria with antibiotics, because treating bacterial colonization when it's not causing any harm leads to bacterial resistance to antibiotics. This is a huge problem not only in the area of UTIs but in conditions such as upper respiratory infections (bronchitis, pneumonia, sinus infections, etc.) where symptoms are caused by viruses, not bacteria, yet antibiotics are given.

## Complicated and Uncomplicated UTI

Another way we classify UTI's is by complicated or uncomplicated. This determines how we treat them. Most UTI's like cystitis, are uncomplicated. The symptoms are familiar to most everyone – painful frequent urination, having a severe urge to go, sometimes pink or bloody urine, multiple trips to the bathroom at night, small amounts of urine voided with a thin intermittent stream, foul-smelling urine, pelvic pain, and pain in the urethra and vagina. The diagnosis is made with what's called a "dipstick" which is placed in a urine specimen that's been properly collected. This method of collection is called a clean catch midstream collection. I'm going to spend a minute on this because as simple a concept as it is, it oftentimes is neglected. When a specimen is not properly collected, the results can be confusing.

When a woman goes to her doctor with symptoms of a UTI, she's told "go to the lab for a UA" (urine analysis). Sometimes (not often enough in my opinion) she's instructed on how to obtain a clean catch midstream UA: "Sit on the toilet with your legs wide apart. Use two fingers of one hand to separate the lips of your vagina so that the urethral opening is exposed. Begin peeing in the toilet. In the middle of the stream, with your other hand holding the specimen container, pee into the specimen container."

The reason we want a midstream urine sample, rather than have you pee into the specimen container right from the start, is that a midstream sample reduces the chances of bacteria from the vagina contaminating the sample, which could lead to a misdiagnosis. So whenever you provide a urine sample, be sure it's a midstream clean catch sample.

What happens to that urine sample, once you've provided it? In the lab, the dipstick is placed into the specimen. The little squares measure several things like blood, protein, and pH levels, as well as nitrites which indicates the presence of bacteria, and "leukocyte esterase" which signals the presence of white blood cells. White blood cells are part of your immune system that help get rid of the bacteria.

The urine is then spun in a centrifuge and examined under the microscope. In acute cystitis, the bacteria and white blood cells can be seen and counted. The urine is then cultured so that whatever bacteria is causing the UTI can be identified. We can also tell which antibiotics are going to be effective against that particular bacteria, and to what degree, and which antibiotics are not likely to work because the bacteria may be resistant to that particular antibiotic. Unfortunately, information regarding sensitivity may not be available for 24-48 hours. What is known immediately, however, is whether or not an infection is present.

Once an infection has been confirmed, you will be started on an antibiotic that is "likely" to work for "the most likely" bug. With simple first time cystitis in women most bacteria are susceptible to several antibiotics. Taking allergies into consideration, trimethoprim-sulfa (Septra DS or Bactrim DS one pill twice a day), nitrofurantoin (Macrodantin 100 mg four times a day), or ciprofloxacin (Cipro 500 mg twice a day) all should work, but may have to be changed depending on bacterial sensitivities. How long you should take the prescribed antibiotic is controversial, ranging from one day to one week. I usually recommend a three day course.

Keep in mind that the antibiotic will kill the bacteria causing the infection, they won't necessarily ease your discomfort immediately. For relief of symptoms, I prescribed Pyridium (an anesthetic for the urinary tract) 100 mg three times a day. If your physician prescribes this medication for you, be forewarned, it will make your urine orange, so don't be alarmed). You should be feeling better within 24-48 hours. If your symptoms don't subside after two days, call your doctor. It's possible that you need a different antibiotic because the bug that's causing your infection may not be sensitive to the antibiotic you are taking. In this case, your physician will switch you to a different antibiotic.

## Recurrent UTIs

If your uncomplicated cystitis has cleared up after antibiotics, but recurs a few weeks or months later, you may need to be on a different antibiotic for a longer course (5-7 days). While it's not unusual to have recurring UTI's within a few months, if it recurs within six months, further evaluation is indicated. Although there are simple reasons for recurrent lower tract infections in women (such as an active sex life, which can cause bacteria to be pushed into the urethra, dehydration, diabetes, constipation, and loss of the protective lining of the bladder), it's necessary to rule out structural abnormalities in either or both kidneys, such as a blocked kidney, or a stone(s). An ultrasound of both kidneys and bladder (before and after voiding) can address the problem of recurrent infections.

The main reason why women get recurrent uncomplicated lower recurrent UTIs (cystitis or bladder infections) has to do with sex and a substance that normally coats the lining of the bladder called a "slippery substance." The technical name for this "Teflon-bladder lining" is glycosaminoglycan, or GAG, layer. This slippery substance is normally present in the bladder and its purpose is to prevent bacteria from sticking to the bladder lining. So even if a pathogen such as e. coli gets pushed into the urethra during sex and ultimately reaches the bladder, if a woman pees after sex, and the slippery substance does its job, the bacteria will simply be peed out. But if you've had an aggressive bacterial infection, the *infection may have temporarily destroyed this layer*. If there is no GAG layer, the bacteria will stick, set up camp, multiply, and result in another infection. It takes about six months for the GAG layer to grow back, which explains how an infection can recur, even with a bug that was sensitive to the original antibiotic. For this reason, if a sexually active woman has more than one infection within a six month period, a daily *small* dose of an antibiotic (usually nitrofurantoin, trimethoprim/sulfa, or trimethoprim alone) for six months can prevent the bacteria from colonizing and therefore prevent another infection while the GAG layer grows back. Another way of managing recurrent uncomplicated cystitis is with a small dose of an antibiotic after sex.

Estrogen also provides some protection against bacterial invasion via the urethra, so when estrogen levels drop following menopause, women lose that added protection. For this reason, elderly post-menopausal women, even those who aren't sexually active, can suffer from recurrent UTI's. The same rules apply as far as the need for an ultrasound of the kidneys and pre and post void (empty) bladder, and suppressive antibiotics. For these women, provided there is no contraindication to taking estrogen, topical estrogen cream applied to the genitalia may help prevent recurrence.

It goes without saying that there are simple things you can do to prevent recurrent cystitis Practice good hygiene. After peeing wipe from top to bottom, front to back and drop the toilet paper in the toilet, if you need to wipe more, get another piece of TP. Wear cotton underwear, drink lots of water. Cranberry juice helps. And (this may not get discussed very often), no anal intercourse.

Not all UTI's are simple and uncomplicated, however. In some cases, a simple urine analysis and culture are insufficient. Let's consider these more complicated urinary tract infections.

## Complicated UTI's in Women

There is a whole list of things that make a UTI in a woman complicated. If there is a known structural abnormality involving the kidneys, ureters, bladder, or urethra, the infection is considered "complicated." Women who get infected with a UTI and who also have GI illnesses such as ulcerative colitis or Crohn's Disease, may develop complicated UTIs, because of an abnormal connection between the GI tract and the urinary tract. Pregnant women who have a UTI are also at increased risk related to not just the health of the pregnant mother, but also to the fetus.

Women who have other medical problems such as diabetes, or who have had a kidney transplant, should be regarded as having a complicated UTI, and be evaluated and possibly treated differently than a healthy woman with uncomplicated cystitis. This usually means imaging (US, CT, or MRI) and possibly a look in the bladder with a scope (cystoscopy). If there is a problem with bladder emptying, the woman should be evaluated for a neurological disease (such as diabetes mellitus, multiple sclerosis, and a variety of other diseases that can possibly cause incomplete bladder emptying). If the organism (bug) causing the UTI is something unusual (something other than the common gram negative bug that cause UTIs like e.coli, klebsiella, proteus, Enterobacter), then the infection should be thought of as complicated. Finally, if there is visible blood in the urine along with the initial UTI, and the blood does not go away after successful antibiotic treatment, that also qualifies as a complicated UTI and you should see a urologist.

## Conclusion

In closing, if you have a UTI, your PCP will treat you with an appropriate antibiotic. If you continue to have UTI's, you might want to see a urologist, who will do whatever tests are necessary to figure out why you got a UTI in the first place. These tests will likely include an ultrasound of your bladder before and after you pee to see how much your bladder holds and how much urine is left in your bladder after you pee, an ultrasound of your kidneys, and possibly cystoscopy to have a look at your urethra and bladder.

# CHAPTER 5

# Everybody Must Get Stones

One of the most common questions I get asked on the golf course, at dinner parties, or anywhere I'm introduced to a group of new people and they learn that I'm a urologist, will inevitably be about kidney stones. "I've had kidney stones about a dozen times," someone will say, "and let me tell you, they're worse than having a baby."

"Sorry to hear that," I'll say, as I try to focus on my golf shot or take a stab at my appetizer. "Are you still getting them?"

"Yeah, my urologist wants to blast them again. What do you think? Should I go ahead and have them blasted?"

"Hard to say," I'll reply as I make my shot or take a bite of my shrimp cocktail. "I'd have to see your medical records and X-rays, but . . ."

Everyone has a story about their kidney stones, or their husband's stones, their wife's stones, their in-law's, or friend's. Sometimes it seems as if each one has a more involved stone story than the one that came before. It's conversations like these that makes me wonder why I didn't choose another profession.

Fortunately, I love my profession, especially when it comes to treating patients with stones. It's really gratifying to relieve a person of horrible pain. Plus, we have all the good toys (lasers, shock wave lithotripsy, ultrasonic lithotripsy) at our disposal to treat stones.

I understand why so many people have questions. Having a kidney stone is usually an unforgettable experience. And they're common. About one in 11 people in the U.S. will have one or more stones in their lifetime, and up to one million people will visit an emergency room for kidney stones. And once you have—or suspect you have—one, you'll want to know what you can do to be rid of it. But all it takes is one Google search to realize there are millions of links to information about kidney stones. Even if a person has the time and ability to sort through this deluge of information, they're just as likely to find misinformation as useful information. While some of this advice is harmless, some of it doesn't work, and some of it can be absolutely harmful. So in this chapter, I want to present you with enough information to make good choices with respect to diagnosis, treatment, and prevention.

## An Overview of Kidney Stones

When we talk about "kidney stones" we're talking about a condition called urolithiasis—Greek for "urinary stones" (loosely translated). These "stones" are concentrations of crystals that can range from the size of a grain of sand up to the size of a tennis ball. I once removed a stone that size from the bladder of a 65 year old man. Stones smaller than 2mm usually don't get stuck, in fact, you may not even know you have one because you'll likely pass it without knowing. Urinary stones can develop almost anywhere in the urinary tract, including the kidneys and the bladder. What's more, they can occur in clusters—I once removed about 30 stones from a single kidney, and over 100 from a bladder!

While stones are common, who gets them varies greatly depending on climate, socioeconomic status, and diet. There are also certain underlying conditions that predispose some people to developing stones. In poorer countries, bladder stones are prevalent in children, largely due to dehydration and insufficient protein. In the United States, stones in children are less common (but they do occur), and more likely to occur in adults between the ages of 30 to 60. Men and women tend to get them in equal numbers, though the gender disparity varies. Stones afflict more people in the South and Southwest, where the incidence is higher during warmer months due to dehydration, when urine is more concentrated. In fact, there is concern that climate change will lead to an increase in kidney stones as a rise in temperature leads to more dehydration. Thus, kidney stones are likely to remain a problem for many.

## Symptoms

How do you know if you have a stone? If you've had one before, you probably know. If you haven't had one before, you may not even know it. If a stone is small (less than 2 or 3 mm), it may not cause symptoms (something we refer to as an asymptomatic stone). If it does cause symptoms, however, those symptoms can include intense pain, nausea, vomiting, fever and/or discolored or bloody urine. Let's take a look at these symptoms one at a time.

Kidney stone pain is usually in the flank, the area in your back just below the ribcage. The pain can be sharp and intense. It can be constant or come in waves. It can move around your side and into your groin and/or genital region. The pain is so distinct that we even have a name for it—renal colic—because it's a pain that will leave you crying.

The nature and character of the pain depends on the size of the stone, where it may be stuck, and if it is stuck, whether it is obstructing the urinary tract. The ureter drains urine from the kidney to the bladder. You have two ureters and each is about a foot long and the diameter of a pencil. So if the stone is tiny (say like a 2 mm grain of sand), it may not cause any pain at all. But a stone larger than 4 mm (a little over 1/8 of an inch) may hurt. As a stone gets closer to the bladder, it's more likely to pass spontaneously, but if it gets stuck in the part of the ureter closest to the kidney, it's less likely to pass spontaneously.

A stone lodged near the kidney that blocks the flow of urine down the ureter will cause increased pressure in the kidney. The pain from this increased pressure can affect your intestines, causing them to shut down. This is called an ileus, and it's effectively a paralysis of your intestines that causes the nausea and vomiting people with obstructing stones often have.

A stone that passes through the urinary tract can irritate the lining of the urinary tract. When this happens, you'll see discolored urine due to blood in the urine, which can appear light pink or dark as red wine. You may also see blood clots, or old blood, which will look like cola or coffee grounds. Sometimes the urine will appear normal to the naked eye, but a urinalysis will show microscopic blood, The urine under the microscope with be filled with red blood cells and sometimes the telltale crystals.

A most concerning symptom of stones is fever. An infected stone can cause fever—these are called struvite stones and are made of magnesium ammonium phosphate and bacteria. You can also have fever from a stone obstructing urine that is stagnant and infected. An obstructing stone and fever can be life threatening. If you have fever and flank pain (with or without discolored urine, nausea and vomiting) you should seek medical attention immediately. It may turn out that you simply have an infected kidney (pyelonephritis, discussed in Chapter 4), it could mean you have an infected stone, or an infection above the obstruction. A severe infection can lead to an abscess in the kidney. The greatest danger is when the infection gets into your bloodstream. This is called "sepsis" (in this case "urosepsis") and can result in shock ("septic shock"), and even death.

Whatever the symptoms, if you have a stone and don't pass it on your own quickly, you're going to need treatment. That treatment will depend on many variables, such as the size of the stone, the location of the stone, what the stone is made of (some stones like those made of uric acid can be dissolved, calcium stones cannot), the presence or absence of obstruction of the urinary tract (from the stone or other causes of obstruction), and whether the stone is single or are there multiple stones.

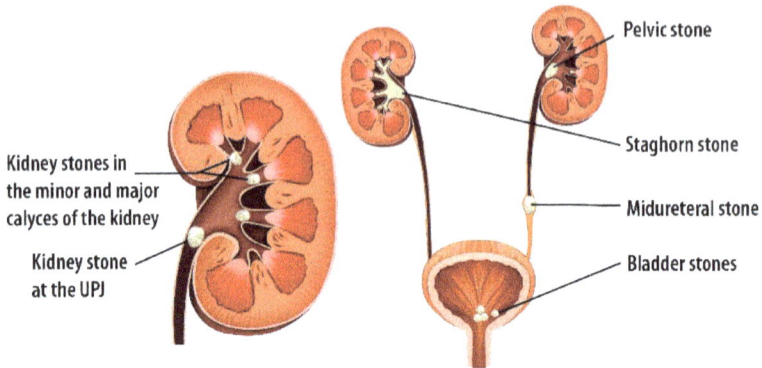

**Possible location of urinary tract stones, also known as _urolithiasis_**

## Treating Urinary Stones

If you listen to your parents or grandparents talk about stones, you're likely to hear about some archaic treatments. We've come a long way in the last four to five decades, and your options for treatment today are in some ways remarkable.

During the first part of my urology residency in the late seventies, we would do a variety of surgical procedures to remove stones from kidneys, ureters (the tubes that drain the kidneys into the bladder), bladders, and urethras. This was before lasers, shock waves, and ultrasonic lithotripters. Everything was done through an incision, what we called "open procedures." It wasn't until the later part of my residency in the early 80s that the subspecialty field of endourology—urological procedures done with minimally invasive techniques primarily through "scopes"—became accepted as a subspecialty within urology. Some older urologists who were comfortable with open procedures to remove stones coined the new practice as "end of urology." Some of them had trouble learning the new techniques, so for them it really was "the end of urology".

In 1985 I attended an AUA (American Urologic Association) meeting and sat in on a talk given by a German urologist who discussed a new technique to break up stones using shockwaves generated outside the body. The anesthetized patient was secured to a chair, which was then lowered into a tub of water. Shockwaves were generated from a device similar to a sparkplug into a thing that looked like a metal bowl. When the shockwaves hit the bowl they were reflected upward. The shape of the reflected shockwave was like an upside down ice cream cone. Using fluoroscopy (x-rays), the stone could be seen, and the special chair was moved to align the stone with the tip of the cone. No incision was involved. The shockwaves, focused on the stone, passed harmlessly through the body. The "sparkplug" generated a new shockwave with each heartbeat of the patient. The maximum force of the shockwave could be varied dependent on how hard the stone was. Thousands of these shockwaves could break up stones into tiny sand-sized particles that would pass harmlessly out of the body in the urine. We sat there listening to this presentation totally astounded. Surgery using mirrors and hocus-pocus? Impossible. 40 years later, this technology, Extracorporeal (outside the body) Shock Wave Lithotripsy (breaking up the stone with shockwaves) is a mainstay treatment for millions of stone formers (though the large bathtub is not used very often). Now there are special tables combined with fluoroscopy that can be moved from one outpatient surgical center to another.

Technological advances continued into the mid and late 1980s. Procedures to treat patients with stones became less invasive, or even noninvasive. Endoscopes used to remove stones from the ureter and kidney went from being rigid to flexible. Optics and cameras improved. We learned how to employ stents to relieve any obstruction and aid in the passing of fragments.

By 1985 I took special courses to learn some of these procedures that did not even exist during my residency a few years earlier. For example, I learned how to do a procedure we referred to as a **PERC**, which stands for percutaneous (through the skin) nephrostolithotomy (nephro—kidney; litho—stone; otomy—removal).

Recall from the anatomy chapter that the kidney is composed of a solid outer part that surrounds an inner or hollow part that collects urine. I used to explain it to my patients by telling them to think of the hollow part or the renal pelvis as a lake surrounded by a land mass (the renal parenchyma or the solid part of the kidney). The 'lake' (renal pelvis) drains into a river (the ureter) that's about a foot long, which then drains into another lake (the bladder). Using fluoroscopy or ultrasound, a needle can be passed through a small one inch incision. The needle is then passed through the solid part of the kidney and into the collecting system and renal pelvis (the lake). Once the collecting system is accessed, a wire can be passed into the renal pelvis and down the ureter. The tissue from the skin to the collecting system (namely muscle and the solid part of the kidney) is dilated to create a "tract" about an inch in diameter. A hollow tube is then inserted into the kidney through the tract. If the stones are smaller than the tube, they are removed intact, and if larger, they are broken up using ultrasound, lasers, or other high-tech toys.

Imagine you are in the ER with kidney stone pain. The ER doctor has just taken a history, done a physical, sent your urine to the lab, and has obtained blood for several tests such as a complete blood count, an evaluation of your electrolytes (sodium, potassium, chloride), kidney function tests, and possibly a serum calcium, phosphorus, and uric acid assessment. As you wait patiently and in agony, s/he finally comes in and says, "I think you may have a kidney stone. I'd like to send you over for a CT scan." (If you are having fever and flank pain and are not in an ER or Urgent Care Clinic where they have rapid access to a CT scanner, but do have access to ultrasound, they might send you for an ultrasound first.)

Before the doctor sends you to get the CT scan, s/he will likely give you something for the pain, and possibly something for nausea. The CT scan will determine whether or not you have a stone and its location, but it probably won't be able to distinguish what type of stone it is, or its composition. That's important information in determining your treatment and how to prevent more stones from forming. (If you've had stones in the past, your physician may assume it's the same type of stone.) For now, let's assume this is your first stone.

If at this point your pain is controlled, you don't have fever, you are able to eat and drink, and your labs are all within normal limits (that is, no sign of infection, your electrolytes are normal, and your kidney function is normal). You may be sent home and an appointment with a urologist will be arranged within 24 hours. (If you have fever or an elevated white count or an obstructing stone, the urologist will be called in immediately and arrange to relieve the obstruction and/or remove the stone. If the ER doctors can't control your pain, or if you are unable to eat or drink, the urologist will likely come in to take care of you and your stone.

But first, let's assume that you are feeling better. You've been in the ER since 3 pm, and it's now 3 am. You've been told that you have a stone stuck in the tube between your kidney and bladder, and you have an appointment to see a urologist the next day. What happens next depends on four things—the size of the stone(s), the location, how much blockage is present, and how you are feeling. After a discussion of those variables, you and your urologist will jointly make a decision about what to do based on the probability of how likely you are to pass the stone on your own. This situation is unique to every patient. There may not be a single right answer, but a urologist with experience in taking care of kidney stone patients usually has a pretty good idea about which ones will pass on their own, and which ones s/he will have to treat. The first decision is, "Should we intervene, or wait and see if it will pass on its own?" Again, this outcome is highly variable, and there is no absolute right way of doing things.

Let's also assume your urologist tells you that you have a greater than 90% chance of passing the stone spontaneously within the next two weeks and gives you a prescription for medicine that will relax the ureteral spasm, which may help the stone pass spontaneously. S/he also sends you home with a urine strainer and instructs you to pee through the strainer until you pass the stone, and tells you to drink lots of water. Your urologist may also assure you that once the stone is in the bladder, it won't hurt when you ultimately pee it out. A 4-5 mm stone is about the size of a match head, and s/he will tell you to look for it in the strainer.

You go home with your strainer and meds and get on the internet to see if there is anything more you can do to help pass the stone. We want you to stay hydrated, but there is no evidence that drinking huge amounts of fluids (more than a gallon or 3.5 liters) helps expel the stone. In fact, drinking huge amounts of water can actually be harmful because it can lower your sodium and potassium levels in your blood. (Later, we'll discuss the importance of water drinking in terms of prevention of new stones from forming.)

While browsing the internet, you're likely to come across claims like, "lemon juice (vitamin C or citric acid) will break down kidney stones." Lemon juice will not dissolve most common (calcium oxalate) stones. However, lots of lemon juice or citrate may help prevent certain types of stones from forming. "Olive oil helps with the flushing process" another site will claim. Again, there's no evidence for that. "Most stones will pass on their own within a few hours to a few days." Again, more misleading information. You know by now that passing a stone depends on the size and the location. Some people are misled by claims that "cranberry juice is good for your urinary tract, so it must be good if you have a kidney stone." While cranberry juice has been shown to be helpful for urinary tract infections, as we'll see soon, it could actually add to the creation of new stones, and it's something we tell recurrent stone formers to *avoid*.

The bottom line is, take your medication, and if all goes well, the stone, depending on size and location, will pass. Be sure to use your strainer. The stone that shows up in the strainer might look like a BB, it may be rough or smooth. It can be black, brown, or yellow. Why save the stone? It's not because it's a keepsake! The reason we want you to save the stone is so we can tell what type it is, which can help determine how to prevent future stones from forming. If more stones do form, your urologist will have a better idea of how to treat you. I'll return to this point at the end of the chapter, but for now, let's consider what happens if you don't pass the stone.

Let's imagine that you've gone home, waited for two weeks, yet still haven't passed the stone. You're tired of peeing through a strainer and you've had intermittent flank pain that's making it impossible to work or think of anything else. You've been back to the ER once, where they repeated the CT scan. You've been taking opioids to control the pain and haven't eaten much. You are sick of it and just want the ordeal to be over. "Get this damn thing out of me!" you beg.

In this situation, the stone is probably stuck. Although blockage can occur anywhere along the course of the ureter, there are three places where larger stones typically get stuck and obstruct: the junction of the kidney (renal pelvis) and ureter  (ureteropelvic junction); two-thirds of the way down the ureter where the ureter crosses the iliac vessels in the pelvis; and the junction of the ureter and bladder (ureterovesical junction)

A general rule is that the larger the stone and/or the closer to the kidney it is, the more likely an intervention is required to relieve the blockage and pain. Stones larger than 6 or 7 mm are much less likely to pass on their own and often become lodged in your urinary tract. If the stone is moderate size (4-7 mm, which is about 1/15 of an inch to a quarter inch), and causing blockage and pain, you might consider a **stent**. Stents are soft plastic tubes about 2 mm in diameter. The center or lumen of the tube is hollow like a straw. There are tiny holes up and down the course of the tube. There are two J shaped curls on each end of the stent. One end curls up in the collecting system of the kidney and the other end curls in the bladder so the stent can't migrate either out of the kidney and down the ureter or conversely out of the bladder and up toward the kidney. Some urologists will place these stents under general anesthesia. Others will place them under local with conscious sedation. Stones of moderate size may pass spontaneously after two weeks of an indwelling stent, which is easily removed under local anesthesia in the office via flexible cystoscopy.

If the stone is larger than 6 mm, a procedure to break the stone up, or remove the stone is likely necessary. Placing a JJ stent before any stone procedure has the advantage of relieving the obstruction and the pain. An added benefit is that the stent passively dilates the ureter, which makes future procedures safer with better outcomes than not having a stent. These benefits are in exchange for possible minor discomfort from the stent. Some patients tolerate stents very well and don't even know that the stent is there, while others can experience bladder discomfort, frequent or painful urination, or possible pain in the kidney with urination. Pain in the kidney with urination while a stent is in place happens because during urination the pressure in the bladder is felt in the kidney since the two are connected by the stent. When you urinate the pressure increases, which can cause discomfort in the kidney. This is not common, and the pain from a stent is usually nowhere near the amount from the stone. However, with a stent there is also the risk of a urinary tract infection.

If your urologist feels that spontaneous passage is unlikely, then there are a variety of techniques designed either to break the stone up into small fragments, sand-like particles, or dust. The instruments designed to break a stone up are passed through a scope. The scope designed to break a stone up in the ureter is called a ureteroscope, and the procedure is called uretroscopic lithotripsy. The ureteroscope is a thin (about 4-5 mm) flexible fiberoptic scope passed through the urethra, then bladder, and then into the ureter. The image from the camera part of the ureteroscope is viewed on a TV monitor. Under vision a variety of thin, flexible laser fibers are passed through the scope. The urologist controls and sets the frequency of the laser impulses and energy that goes through the fiber that results in breaking of the stone into small particles or dust. Following the procedure, a JJ stent may be necessary for a week or two to allow the swelling in the ureter to go down and also for any small fragments to pass.

Another technique for breaking up a stone in the ureter is the procedure I learned to do in the mid-eighties—**Shock Wave Lithotripsy.** The shockwaves are exactly (within 1 or 2 mm) focused on the location of the stone. Every time your heart beats another shockwave is triggered. The urologist can vary strength or intensity of the shockwave depending on where the stone is, the size, and whether it appears particularly hard. Shockwaves break the stone into small fragments. The larger the stone, the bigger the fragments and the larger the stone, the more shocks are needed. Usually, a double J stent is placed prior to the procedure, which both aids the urologist in locating the stone with fluoroscopy (x-rays) and helps the fragments pass once the stent is removed (though small fragments can also pass with the stent in place).

Stone too large to pass

Ultrasound shock waves

Smaller pieces pass
out of the body in urine

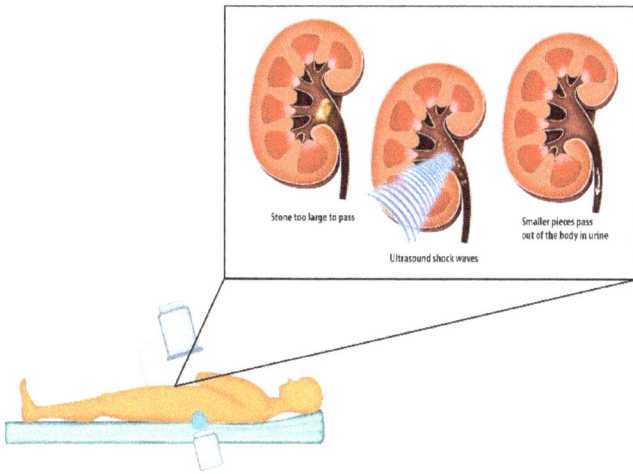

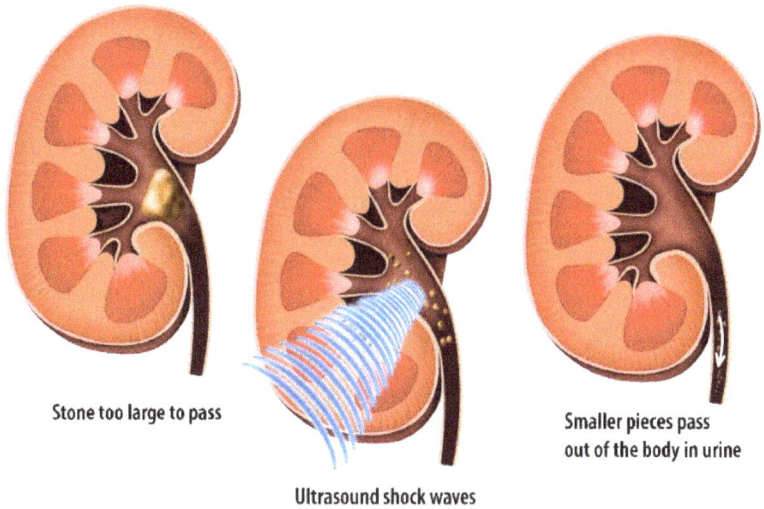

# Extracorporeal Shock Wave Lithotripsy – ESWL

Either of these procedures— ureteroscopic lithotripsy or **Extracorporeal Shock Wave Lithotripsy (ESWL)**—can be done both for stones in the ureter or in the actual kidney. The decision to do one or the other procedure is a matter of weighing risks and benefits. The two procedures share similar risks and benefits, but there are also a different set of risks and potential complications associated with each. Depending on the size, location, and how hard the stone is, ureteroscopic lithotripsy (usually with a laser) may have an advantage over ESWL in getting you "stone free;" however, since ureteroscopic lithotripsy is more invasive than ESWL, the risk of injuring the ureter or kidney for example, may be greater. On the other hand, ESWL has a greater chance of leaving residual fragments. This discussion may vary from one urologist to the next based on experience, personal bias, and what tools the urologist has available. You may choose to have the less invasive (ESWL) procedure in exchange for the possibility of needing a second ESWL for residual fragments, or you may opt for ureteroscopy, because even though the risks may be higher, there's a better chance of you being stone free after one procedure.A good shared decision making discussion with your urologist often helps with this decision. Finally, if the stone is small enough, or if the ureter has been dilated, the stone can be removed intact using a "stone basket" passed through the ureteroscope.

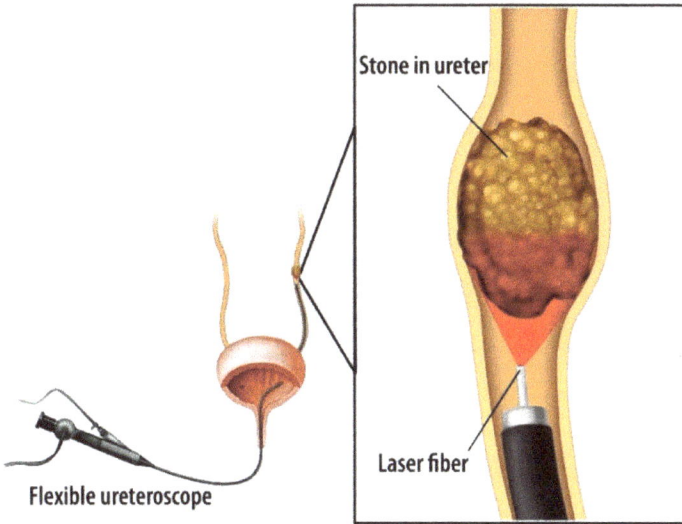

**Ureteroscopic ureterolithotomy using flexible ureteroscope and a variety of different lasers that turn the stone into tiny fragments, sand, or dust.**

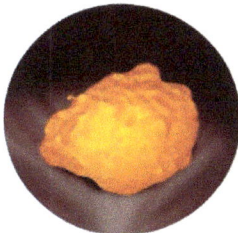

Stone

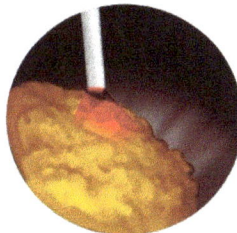

Laser fiber

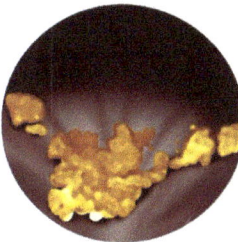

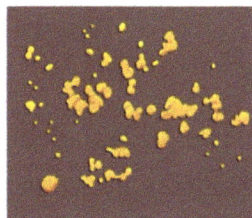

## Stone fragments after laser lithotripsy

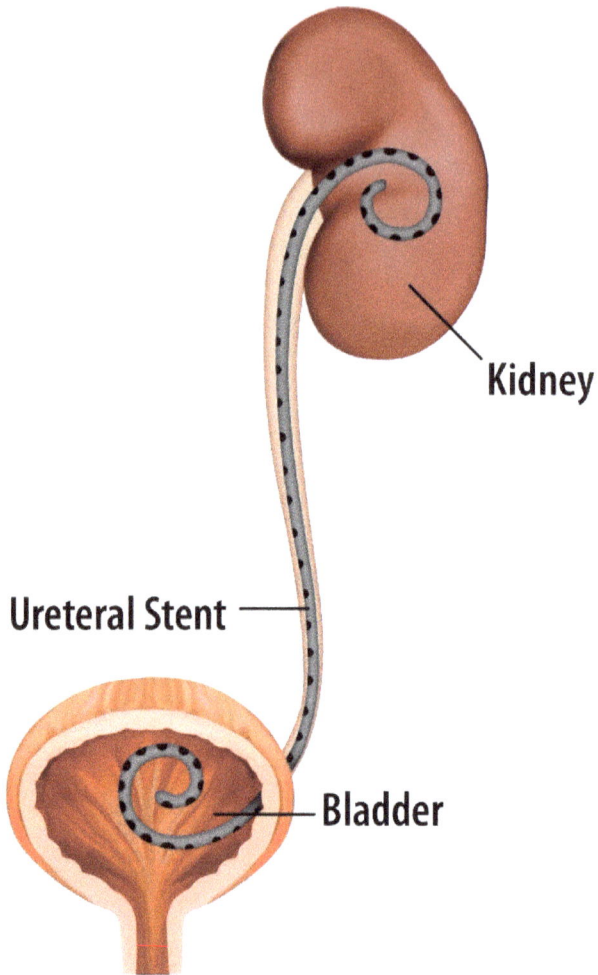

**Double J stent**

There are two instances in which a different intervention is necessary. Sometimes the stone is so stuck, and the swelling is so severe that the urologist can't relieve the obstruction. Another situation is when there is a significant obstruction with a severe infection, sometimes with a high fever, sometimes even with septic shock. In such cases, a radiologist can pass a nephrostomy tube into the kidney using ultrasound and/or x-rays. The tube drains the kidney and the infected, obstructed urine, and allows the doctors to relieve pressure in the kidney. Once the patient is stable, the infection treated, the shock and sepsis resolved, the urologist can then address the stone(s) that caused all the problems.

## Stones in the Kidneys

Thus far we've mainly been discussing stones in the ureter. Stones can form in the kidney and remain there without causing any symptoms, even if quite large. On the other hand, if the stones in the kidney block the flow of urine, it's going to hurt. Stones in the kidney can also cause bleeding and infection.

Stones in the kidney can be treated in a similar fashion to stones in the ureter—with ureteroscopy or ESWL. If the stones are large (greater than 1.0 cm for some urologists), multiple, in the lower portion of the kidney, or "trapped" in a portion of the kidney, then the fragments created after ESWL have a low probability of passing. In this case, ESWL is not a good idea. Similarly, if the stone is in a tough place to get to with a ureteroscope, you may want to consider a different procedure. The same holds true for very large (> 2 cm) and multiple stones. It's not that ureteroscopy in these circumstances can't be done, it's just that the procedure could take hours and you still may not be stone free at the end. An alternative minimally invasive procedure in these cases is a percutaneous (through the skin) nephrosto (through the kidney) lithotomy (remove the stone) or PNL.

Prior to finishing my residency in 1982, procedures for extremely large and stag horn calculi (large, branched kidney stones, sometimes infected) were done via a foot-long open incision. Once the kidney was exposed, we had to bivalve it like opening a clam (anatrophic nephrolithotomy) or open the renal pelvis (pyelolithotomy) in order to extract the large stone(s). For multiple stones in the kidney, we did a different open procedure called a "coagulum pyelolithotomy" in which we injected a solution that would form a cast-like jelly clot around the stones, which we then removed. Percutaneous Nephrostolithotomy (PNL) has rendered those invasive open procedures virtually obsolete.

If you and your urologist decide a PNL is best, you are put under general anesthesia. A catheter is placed in the ureter. Radiographic dye (to which is added a blue dye called methylene blue) is infused through the catheter in the ureter. You are positioned face down or on your side on the operating table. A one-inch incision is made in the back and a needle is inserted into the kidney under fluoroscopic or ultrasound guidance. Once the needle enters the kidney, a blue dye is infused into the kidney. A wire is advanced through the needle and guided down the ureter. A special balloon-dilating catheter is passed over the wire into the kidney, the tract is dilated to about an inch in diameter and a hollow tube is passed over the balloon dilating catheter and into the kidney. Through that tube, a rigid or flexible endoscope is passed and the stone is removed whole (if it's less than 1.0 cm) or broken into smaller fragments using either ultrasound (like a hollow jack hammer with suction) or lasers. Once all of the stones are removed, a nephrostomy tube is put into place in case there is post-op bleeding, residual stones in the kidney, or obstructing stones in the ureter. The following day, a CT scan is done to be sure all of the stone and fragments have been removed. If not, the nephrostomy tube enables us to look back in the kidney a few days later and remove whatever is left. If the kidney is "clean," the nephrostomy tube is clamped and then removed the next day and you are discharged home.

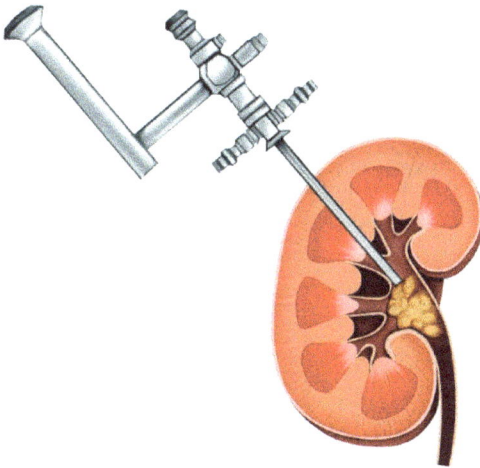

Percutaneous Nephrostolithotomy done through a 1" incision in the back through a rigid nephroscope for a large stone in the renal pelvis. A variety of different energy sources (ultrasound, lasers, etc) are used to break the stone (s) up.

## PNL

In my opinion, PNLs are technically demanding. The procedure can be difficult for many reasons, and complications include bleeding, incomplete removal of the stones, infection, injury to the kidney, and even a collapsed lung (pneumothorax). So you want to be sure that if your urologist is recommending this procedure that s/he has discussed the alternatives and potential complications of all the procedures that are possible. And you want to be sure that the person who is doing the PNL has significant training, experience, and success with the procedure. Don't be afraid to ask. An experienced and skilled urologist will have no trouble answering any questions you may have.

## Prevention

If you've ever recovered from a kidney stone, you've likely made it through level one of Dante's journey through stone hell. Congratulations. Hopefully as you read this you are stone free—that is, there are no stones anywhere in your urinary tract. The stones have all been removed or you've passed them. What comes next is important because for the most common calcium containing stones, you have a 50% chance of getting another stone within five years. Most people do *not* want to have to go through this again. The risk of recurrent stones is even higher if you have other medical conditions like gout, hyperparathyroidism, obesity, or diabetes.

After you've passed the stone or have had the stone successfully treated, your urologist will send the stone or fragments to a lab for analysis to learn what type of stone it is. Several lab tests will also have already been done or will be done to rule out some of the medical conditions that predispose people to forming stones. Knowing these two bits of information—the type of stone, and any underlying medical condition predisposing you to developing stones—will aid your urologist in helping you to prevent a recurrence.

When talking about prevention, stone type is a good place to start. Since calcium oxalate is the most common type stone affecting 75% of first time stone formers, we will start our discussion with that.

Stones are basically crystals. About three-quarters of stones are made of calcium, either calcium oxalate or calcium phosphate. A more rare calcium stone is calcium carbonate. The common calcium oxalate stone can be made up of monohydrate or dihydrate crystals. Monohydrate stones are typically harder than others, which means they are harder to break up with the variety of energy sources your urologist will use (lasers, ultrasound, or shockwaves). **These calcium stones cannot be dissolved with diet or medication.**

About 15% of stones are **uric acid stones**. Uric acid stones are generally softer than calcium stones and do not show up on regular x-rays. They are seen on ultrasound, CT scans and MRI. Because uric acid is a byproduct of an organic compound called purine, if you have uric acid stones you'll want to avoid foods high in purine—beef, poultry, eggs, fish and organ meats. Thus, unlike calcium oxalate stones, there are dietary measures and medications you can take to help dissolve the stones. People with gout can form uric acid stones, and there are medications available to lower uric acid in the blood (allopurinol), which helps both gout and prevents new uric acid stones.

Another even less common stone is called a **struvite stone.** Struvite stones comprise about ten percent of all stones, and are made of magnesium, ammonium, and phosphate. Struvite stones are associated with urinary tract infections. The bacteria causing the infection produce an enzyme called urease, which splits urea to produce ammonia. As the urine becomes less acidic or more alkaline, the urinary tract becomes a favorable environment for the formation of struvite crystals.

There is an inherited disorder that makes prevention crucial. Cystinuria is a rare form of inherited stone disease seen in one of 10,000 people. Cysteine and cystine are amino acids containing sulfur. Like all amino acids found in blood, they are filtered by the kidney and then reabsorbed by the kidney and returned to the bloodstream. People with this inherited disorder can't reabsorb cysteine or cystine and since the two molecules are not soluble, crystals and stones form. The less hydrated a person is, the greater a stone will form (which is true of all stones).

People diagnosed with cystine stones typically are recurrent stone formers. If you are one of these people, you would most likely benefit from a consultation with a dietician to be sure you are doing everything you can to prevent more stones. It will also benefit your family and offspring to seek genetic counseling.

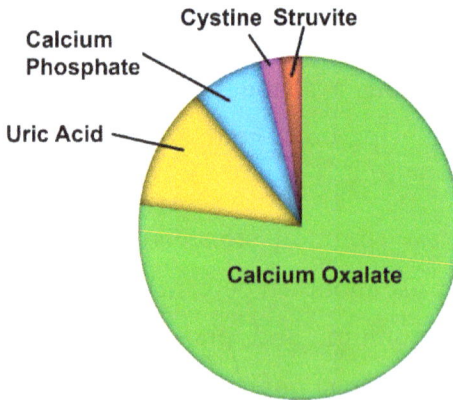

**Not all stones are calcium oxalate. Note that uric acid and cystine stones are not seen on routine x-rays, but are seen on CT.**

Now that you get a picture of the different stone types it's time to do something to keep them from coming back. The most common stone, calcium oxalate, forms because the urine is too concentrated, which allows the crystals to grow. While drinking lots of water won't necessarily help you to pass a stone, staying hydrated will help prevent new stones from forming. Staying hydrated throughout the day is the most important thing you can do, and you can start doing it now. You should drink enough water so that your urine is clear to light colored, which means at least eight glasses a day. I recommend the "water drinking rule of two" to my patients—two 8 ounce glasses first thing in the morning, a glass with each meal, a glass 2 hours after each meal, and 2 glasses at bedtime. That's 10 glasses a day. Most people who drink this much water will have to get up at least once a night to pee. Have another glass then. Adding lemon or lime to your water may also help, because the citrate in the lemon or lime juice prevents calcium oxalate precipitation in the urine. Lemonade can significantly increase urinary citrate and be beneficial in reducing recurrent stones. Finally, an over-the-counter product you can buy on Amazon called Moonstone increases urinary citrate and has been shown to be beneficial. But beware, many supplements being promoted in the media and on the internet claim to prevent recurrent stone formation. They don't.

Another dietary factor that increases the risk of stones forming is a diet high in animal protein. Throughout my practice of over thirty years, few vegetarians or vegans came to me with stones, which should tell you something about calcium oxalate stone prevention. Diets high in grains, nuts, seeds, legumes, and tuberous vegetables further decrease the risk. There is evidence that in older adults, magnesium, potassium and increased fluid intake reduced risk, whereas intake of Vitamin C increased the risk.

The next thing you'll want to do is limit your salt (sodium or Na+) intake. Salt is everywhere and in everything, so check labels. Processed foods, takeout foods, and any food served in a restaurant tends to be high in salt. Replace salt with spices and/or lemon for flavor. Excretion of Na+ and calcium are linked, so by restricting salt, you will decrease the amount of calcium in the urine. Your goal should be no more than two grams of sodium a day.

Some patients assume limiting the amount of calcium and calcium containing foods in their diet prevents new stone formation. It's rational to think limiting dietary calcium will decrease the amount of calcium in the urine, and thus prevent more stones from forming. However, the concentration of oxalate in the urine is a more important determinant of recurrent stone formation than the concentration of calcium. A lot of **dietary oxalate results in increased oxalate concentration in the urine, which, behind hydration, salt, and protein, is the fourth most important factor in recurrent ca-ox stones.**

Calcium oxalate is a salt. If you ingest enough calcium, that calcium binds to oxalate in the gut and prevents GI absorption of some of the oxalate. The calcium oxalate in the gut gets absorbed a lot less from the gut than free oxalate, so you poop oxalate bound to calcium. It stands to reason then that it's more important to reduce dietary oxalate, than it is to restrict calcium. In fact, you should not restrict dietary calcium at all.

But we do want you to watch your oxalate intake. Foods high in oxalate include spinach and other leafy green vegetables, soy, almonds, potatoes, beets, navy beans, raspberries, and more. This is one time that I'd recommend Googling "foods high in oxalate" and see if you are ingesting one of the many culprit foods high in oxalate. Some of these foods high in oxalate have health benefit, so you should not eliminate them entirely, just limit them. A low oxalate diet combined with proper hydration is preferable. I recently had a friend who endured a three month ordeal with a calcium oxalate stone. After it was resolved we talked about his diet to which he replied, "my wife and I eat spinach almost every night."

In short, I would instruct my patients on the "five pillars" for reducing calcium oxalate stones—drink a lot of water throughout the day, limit salt intake, eat minimal animal protein (which includes dairy products, especially ones high in animal fat such as butter and cream), watch your dietary oxalate, and don't decrease your calcium intake.

## Prevention of Calcium Oxalate Stones

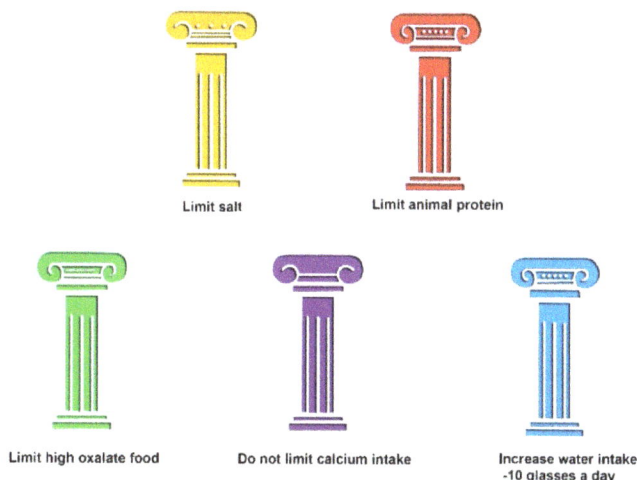

Limit salt

Limit animal protein

Limit high oxalate food

Do not limit calcium intake

Increase water intake
-10 glasses a day

# 5 pillars of calcium oxalate stone prevention

Because diet and hydration are so important in stone disease, I had all of my patients (first timers *and* frequent flyers with recurrent stones) keep a diet diary for two weeks. I'd request that they write everything down, the time of day that they ate or drank, pills/medication, and the amount. From the diary I'd get an idea of their hydration habits, and I'd be able to see if there was anything in the diet to cause stone formation.

What about cranberry juice? Most people assume that cranberry juice is good for your kidneys and urinary tract. This is true if you are prone to urinary tract infections, but it's not true if you've had calcium oxalate stones, because cranberry juice has a lot of oxalate in it. Similarly, grapefruit juice has also been associated with a high risk of stone formation.

Large amounts of vitamin C will cause calcium oxalate stones to form, so you don't want to take vitamin C supplements. Most people get enough vitamin C in the diet, so there is no need to take extra. Besides, large amounts of vitamin C has never been shown to prevent colds or make colds go away faster, despite the myths that they do.

We've just been talking about first time calcium oxalate stone formers. If this is your second time around with a calcium oxalate stone, or if the stone analysis shows a stone type other than calcium oxalate, the evaluation becomes a little more involved. No matter what kind of stone you have, since the goal is to keep you stone free, we will want to dig a deeper and do what's called a "metabolic work up" in addition to the standard history, physical exam, blood tests and diet diary. A metabolic work up is basically collecting urine over 24 hours and measuring important chemicals and compounds within the urine

- pH or the amount of acid in urine, sodium, potassium, chloride, citrate, oxalate, calcium, uric acid, and creatinine.

Putting all the variables together will help us decide if you could benefit from more treatment in addition to the five pillars of prevention. A metabolic work-up can be done by a urologist specializing in stones, or it can be done by a primary care provider with an interest and expertise in stone prevention, or it can be done by an endocrinologist. There are additional medications that may be beneficial if you are a recurrent stone former. And there are several promising therapies (probiotics, gene modification) on the horizon.

## Bladder Stones

Bladder stones are more common in men over 50 because they form in stagnant urine, which can happen with men who have an enlarged prostate, but they do occur in women. Urine that stays in the bladder allows the crystals to get together and form a stone. Stones can also occur in an out-pouching in the bladder called a "diverticulum" (an abnormal sac or out pouching). They also form in both men and women who don't empty their bladders because of nerve damage (diabetes, spinal cord injury, or multiple sclerosis for example). Bladder stones can be single or multiple and range in size from the size of a pencil eraser to a tennis ball. They are frequently associated with a urinary tract infection. Most bladder stones are treated through the urethra using lasers, ultrasound, or an instrument I favored called a "lithoclast" (combination of ultrasound and pneumatic energy). It's important to not only remove the stone but treat the cause of the stagnant urine.

## Conclusion

If you've made it this far, this may be your first journey through stone hell, or you may have been there before, maybe more than once. As you know, having a stone can be a dreadful experience, and you are faced with many decisions: should I wait and see if the stone passes, or should I go for a procedure to remove it? If I chose to have a procedure, should I agree to have the one that will get rid of the stone, or should I opt for a less invasive procedure that may leave residual fragments which could require another procedure? What caused my stone(s) and what can I do to keep them from coming back? If you are currently plagued with a stone sitting somewhere in your urinary tract, you'll want to work with your urologist to make a shared decision about what to do about it. You have options, and the options should be explained to you with respect to risks and benefits of each potential procedure. We have many tools to help you through this hellish experience, and rest assured, these tools (lasers, ESWL, ultrasonic lithotripsy) have made modern day treatment of stones much better than it was 30 or 40 years ago. "Cutting for stone" very rarely happens these days. Once the acute episode is resolved, hopefully you can appreciate how critical hydration and other dietary measures are for prevention. Together you and your urologist will get you out of a painful experience you never want to have again.

# CHAPTER 6

# Bladder Cancer

If you are reading this chapter, you or someone you love probably has bladder cancer. In 2022 there will be over 80,000 new cases of bladder cancer in the U.S. That represents about 4.25% of new cases of cancers of all types. There will be over 17,000 deaths from bladder cancer, which represents 2.8% of all cancer deaths. Although men with bladder cancer outnumber women three to one, women do develop cancer of the bladder. Fortunately, bladder cancer has a high rate of survival. If you are diagnosed with bladder cancer (all types, grades, and stages) your five-year survival rate is 77% (2012-2018).

The bladder is a hollow organ that holds urine. There are three layers to the bladder wall—the lining or mucosa, which is a very thin layer of cells called "transitional cells," a layer of muscle (smooth muscle as opposed to skeletal muscle) and a covering outer layer called serosa. The lining layer of transitional cell mucosa extends from the bladder and lines both ureters, and the lining of the hollow portion of the kidneys where urine begins to collect before being transported down to the bladder via the ureters. Each ureter and the part of the urethra that goes through the urethra is also lined with transitional cells.

When this transitional cell layer starts to grow out of control to form a tumor, it's called transitional cell cancer. There are benign tumors of the bladder, but these are less common, and the pathologist can tell the difference. Almost all (95%) bladder cancers are transitional cell cancers. Other bladder cancers are squamous cell cancers (3%) and adenocarcinomas (2%). Transitional cell cancers also occur in the ureters and the kidneys.

If you smoke cigarettes you are four times likely to develop bladder cancer. If you smoked previously, you are two times more likely to get bladder cancer compared to someone who has never smoked. The risk is the same for male and female smokers. Cigarette smoke carcinogens get into the bloodstream, and then are excreted in urine. The urine containing the carcinogens sit in the bladder for hours in-between void, so it's no wonder smokers get bladder cancer. Other carcinogens like aromatic amines (found in hair dyes, diesel exhaust, and more) cause a variety of cancers including bladder cancer. Arsenic and aromatic hydrocarbons (in coal, gasoline, coal tar pitch and asphalt) also play a role in causing bladder cancer.

I had several patients who worked as hairdressers with bladder cancer. A drug called cyclophosphamide which is used to treat lymphomas and leukemias among other things predisposes people to bladder cancer, as does a type of bladder infection with a bug called schistosomiasis, which is a parasite found in the Middle East, Africa, Asia, and parts of South America (this may present as squamous cell cancer of the bladder). Transitional cells cancers are more common in developed industrialized countries compared to poor countries where squamous cell and adenocarcinoma are more common. And external radiation to the pelvic area increases the risk of getting bladder cancer. In short, we are exposed to a number of carcinogens that may lead, over time, to bladder cancer.[*1]

Let's say you are a 60 year old woman who without warning or symptoms and you see blood in the toilet after urinating. You call your primary care provider, and after determining the blood did not come from your vagina (it's been 25 years since you've had a period), s/he schedules you for a CT urogram to be followed by an appointment with a urologist. The urologist will do a history and physical, looking for clues as to what may be causing the blood in your urine. You explain that you have no pain anywhere, and that you are urinating normally. But your urine is beet red and when s/he looks at it under the microscope there are sheets of red blood cells only, no sign of infection, and no crystals that may indicate a stone. Maybe the CT scan shows a tumor in the bladder, maybe not. Your exam is normal. The urologist then says, "Let's take a look in your bladder and see where the blood may be coming from." So how is that done?

---

[1] 'In Portland there is a fairly large community of Ukrainians. For whatever reason, perhaps due to my ability to speak a little Russian, three of these Ukrainians (all men) were referred to see me for gross blood in their urine. When I asked, "Where were you during the Chernobyl accident?" the answers were revealing. One drove a supply truck in and out of the accident site, the other two were downwind. All three were smokers. And all three had high grade bladder cancers. Eleven years after the accident, the incidence of bladder cancer in the region went from 26/100,000 to 36/100,000 https://www.ncbi.nlm.nih.gov/pmc/articles/PMC5926045/. Of course, this is a much more complicated discussion now almost 40 years after the accident, but the fact remains that the incidence of bladder cancer rose significantly among those exposed to the radiation.

Cystoscopy is an outpatient procedure done with local anesthetic. It's not as bad as you might imagine. Xylocaine (Novocain) jelly is first squirted into the urethra. The longer the Xylocaine jelly stays in the urethra, the better it works (the urologist will leave it in for minimum 10 minutes and probably go do something else while you patiently wait). A flexible cystoscope is threaded into the urethra. There are three channels that make up the cystoscope: one for sterile water that flows through a channel; another for the fiber optic camera at the end of the scope; and a third to pass small 2mm wires or instruments. The fiberoptic lens/camera feeds into a monitor, so you can watch the whole procedure on TV.

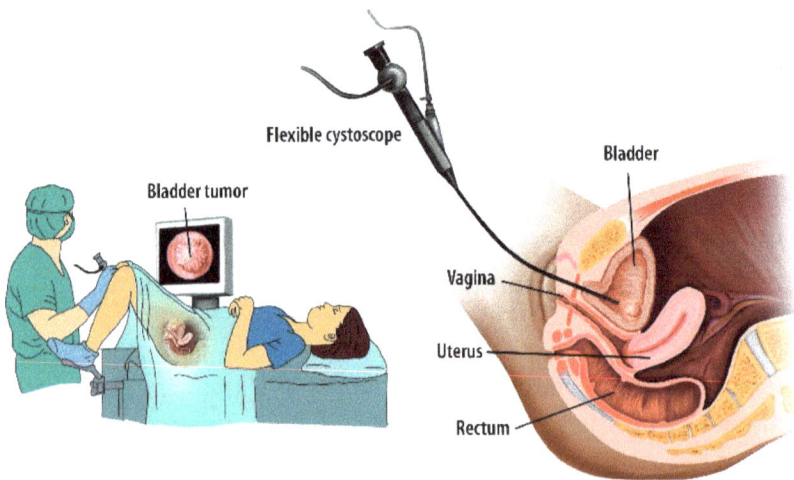

Flexible cystoscopy to diagnose hematuria caused by bladder tumor

## Bladder Tumor

The urologist look closely within the bladder for any abnormal growths. S/he will examine where the tubes draining the kidneys, the ureters, enter. These openings are called "ureteral orifices" and are situated on the floor of the bladder on a triangular shaped part of the bladder called the trigone. If a tumor is found, its location with respect to the ureteral orifices is important as you will see. If no abnormal growth is found, then s/he has effectively ruled out bladder cancer, provided there are no malignant cells noted on a microscopic examination of the urine called urine cytology. The visible blood in the urine is still without an explanation though, so the urologist will want to examine the urinary tract - the ureters and internal collecting system of the kidneys - for a source for the bleeding. If, on the other hand, a bladder tumor is found, your doctor will tell you that you probably have bladder cancer. We have not yet come to the Shared Decision Making part yet, because under most circumstances the next step is to remove the tumor and look at it under the microscope.

The urologist will explain the procedure called a TURBT which stands for "transurethral resection of bladder tumor." Under general or spinal anesthesia, a scope is placed into the bladder. Using saline irrigation and bipolar energy (because it's safer than water and monopolar energy), the tumor is removed and the area from where the tumor is removed is cauterized. Several biopsies of the bladder lining are taken, and the biopsy sites are cauterized. The tissue is sent to a pathologist. Depending on the size of the tumor and whether or not there are multiple tumors, the procedure usually takes 15-60 minutes. A catheter is placed and may be removed in the recovery room before you go home, or one or two days later, depending on the extent of the resection. This is step 1, but that doesn't mean you are out of the woods yet.

Once the pathology report is available, you'll go back to the urologist's office in a few days to discuss the next steps. Prior to that discussion, it's helpful to know something about cancer of the bladder.

Transitional Cell Cancer (TCCA) is *graded* much like other cancers, by the appearance of the cells and the way the cells are arranged. Grades 1, 2, and 3, correspond to the appearance under the microscope and correlate with how fast the cancer is growing, and how likely the tumor is to grow outside the bladder and/or metastasize. Think of transitional cell cancers as either "high grade" (fast growing and likely to spread) or "low grade" (slow growing, unlikely to spread).

Like cancer of the kidney, the TNM staging system is used for bladder cancer. Recall T stands for tumor—the size and whether it's grown outside the bladder into the surrounding tissues; N stands for spread to lymph nodes; and M stands for metastasis.

To determine the T stage, the urologist will review the imaging studies and pathology report. Specifically, the pathologist will state whether the tumor has spread into the muscle layer or not.

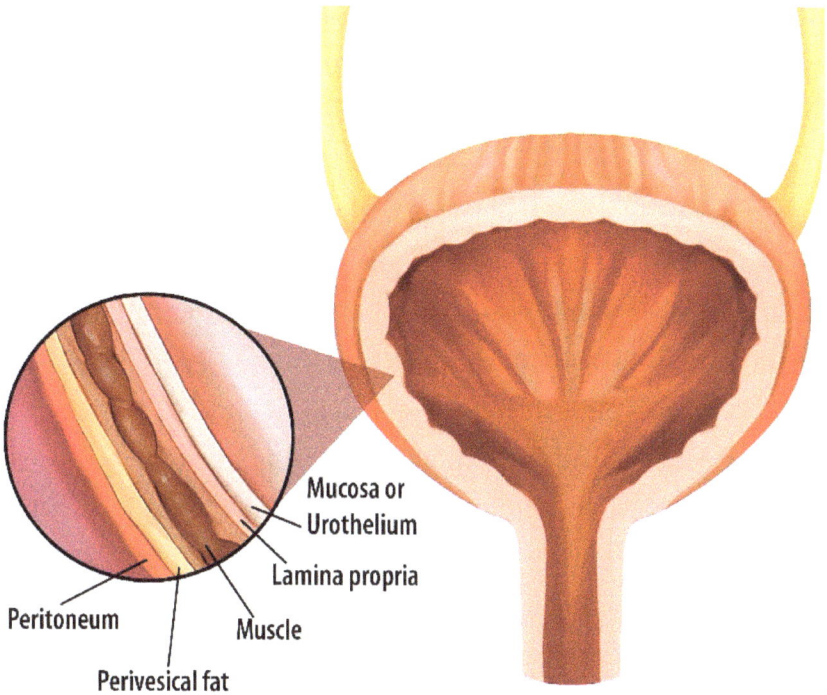

Mucosa or
Urothelium

Lamina propria

Peritoneum

Muscle

Perivesical fat

## Layers of bladder wall

The TCCA will either be non-muscle invasive (NMIBC, non-muscle invasive bladder cancer) or muscle invasive (MIBC, muscle invasive bladder cancer). Let's assume you have a non-muscle invasive tumor. Following the TURBT you are urinating clear urine without problems. Your prognosis depends on the grade of the tumor, the size of the tumor, if there were multiple tumors, or if there are other abnormalities (variant histology) on the biopsies. Overall, for even for high grade NMIBC the prognosis is good with survival between 70% and 85% at 10 years. It's even better for low-grade well differentiated disease. The unfortunate thing is that 70% of TCCAs that are NMIBC will recur, and thus require more treatment. Depending on grade, 5-

25% of NMIBC will progress to muscle invasive cancer despite multiple resections, chemotherapy, or immunotherapy instilled into the bladder. Rates of recurrence and progression correspond to whether the tumor is high or low grade, the presence of CIS (carcinoma in situ, a pathologic diagnosis of a flat tumor that is very aggressive), the T stage, and whether the tumors are multiple or solitary. In other words, bladder cancers are heterogeneous, and every situation needs to be uniquely addressed with the goals of preventing progression, loss of bladder, or loss of life.

After you've made it through step 1 (diagnosis) and step 2 (removal by resection, grading, and staging by pathology) you'll go on to step 3 for non-muscle invasive bladder cancer. Unlike Steps 1 and 2 which are the same for most everyone with NMIBC, step 3 can be extremely variable for each person. It depends on how the stage, grade, and other factors predict risk of progression and recurrence. Your risk of progression is either low, intermediate or high. If you are at low risk of recurrence and/or progression you will undergo cystoscopy every three months for the first year, every six months for the second year, and every year thereafter. If you have a recurrence, however, it's back to step 1.

For intermediate and high risk cancers the follow-up and surveillance are variable and more involved. If there is what's called "variant histology" present, the pathologist will note that in his report. Variant histology is the appearance of cells other than the standard transitional cancer cells. If you have variant histology, you immediately go into the high risk group, and there are multiple options that other high risk patients have, plus the option of partial or total removal of the bladder (discussed below). The risks and benefits of all treatment and surveillance options should be discussed with your urologist.

Immunotherapy and chemotherapy instilled into the bladder (intravesical therapy) work to prevent progression and recurrence in patients with intermediate and high risk disease. Immunotherapy is done with an agent called BCG. The chemotherapeutic agents are Mitomycin C and Gemcitabine. Sometimes these chemotherapeutic agents are introduced into the bladder immediately post operatively (after the original or subsequent resections) through a catheter.

BCG stands for Bacillus Calmette-Guérin. It is a live bacteria similar to the tuberculosis bug, but it doesn't cause an infection. When BCG is in contact with the bladder lining cells, it stimulates the body's immune system to seek out and kill cancer cells. Initial treatments are usually done in the urologist's office once a week for six weeks. During the treatment, your urologist will insert a catheter into your bladder, and inject the BCG through the catheter. Some protocols require maintenance therapy which is done every three months for a year and requires three weekly treatments during those three month intervals.

If there is no visible tumor on follow up cystoscopy, the urologist will want to make sure there is no cancer in the ureters or lining of the kidneys. After initial resection and staging, if blood in the urine persists, and there is no recurrence in the bladder, tumor markers in the urine and urine cytology (a "pap smear" of the urine) can be helpful in pointing toward the possibility of TCCA in the ureters or kidneys. Your urologist will have this in mind as s/he continues to monitor your cancer. Finally, there are newer methods available called "Blue Light Cystoscopy" and "Cxbladder" that have been shown to improve detection of bladder cancer that may not be seen on conventional white light cystoscopy.

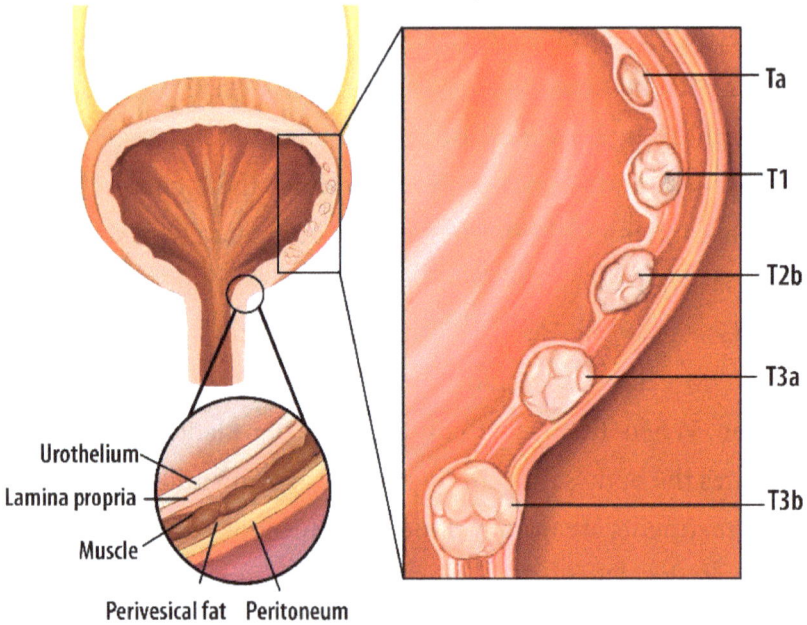

**Stages of bladder cancer. Non-muscle invasive Ta and T1, muscle invasive T2 and T3.**

After Step 1, if the pathology shows tumor has grown into the muscle layer of the bladder, the rules change. This is called muscle invasive bladder cancer, MIBC (stage T2 and T3). Twenty-five percent of patients with bladder cancer will have muscle invasive disease. The risk of progression and metastases is high, so if your cancer has invaded the smooth muscle layer of the bladder, it's serious. If the cancer is invading muscle but confined to the bladder, the five year survival rate is 70% (that means 30% of people will not survive five years, even if the cancer is confined to the bladder and treated). If the cancer has spread to lymph nodes in the pelvis or adjacent organs, the five year survival rate drops to 38%, and if there are distant metastases, the survival rate is less than 10%. Sadly, these statistics have not significantly changed over several decades, but with a team approach to your treatment, you will enhance your chances of beating bladder cancer. You, along with your urologist, an oncologist, and a radiation therapist are part of the team. There are numerous treatment options, again depending on your particular grade and stage, and your life preferences definitely need to be taken into consideration. It's here that a Shared Decision Making Discussion is helpful.

Upon learning that you have MIBC, your urologist will want to further stage the cancer to see if has grown beyond the confines of the bladder, involves adjacent organs, tissue, lymph nodes, bones, or if you have distant spread to distant organs (such as lungs or liver). For this s/he will order a CT of your chest, abdomen, and pelvis (or an MRI), along with a bone scan. A variety of blood tests will be done to further assess your condition, with particular attention to your kidney and liver function.

Once the staging work-up is finished, you will know whether you have metastases. Then, you will discuss your options. Let's assume that the muscle invasive bladder cancer is still confined to the bladder. In other words, based on imaging and blood tests, there is no obvious spread to lymph nodes, no spread to bone, and no distant metastases. Guidelines for treating this disease have evolved during years of research and clinical studies with the goals of improving survival, while at the same time maintaining quality of life.

It used to be that the standard of care for non-metastatic muscle invasive bladder cancer was to proceed as soon as possible with radical cystectomy (removal of the bladder) along with removal of pelvic lymph nodes. The current recommendation, however, for patients in whom the cancer has not spread beyond the bladder or in lymph nodes, is adjuvant chemotherapy (chemo given *before* removal of the bladder). If the cancer is outside the bladder and/or in lymph nodes, a radical cystectomy may be done, and the chemotherapy is given after the surgery.

Finally, if you do have distant metastases, the first course of therapy is chemotherapy. Your response to chemotherapy (the stage of the cancer after chemotherapy) and your overall state of health determines the next steps, which include surgery, radiation, more or different chemotherapy. This area of oncology is changing so rapidly due to the new "check point inhibitor" drugs that by the time you read this, whatever I write will be outdated, so we'll just leave it at that.

## Radical Cystectomy and Urinary Diversion

A radical cystectomy in a woman consists of complete removal of the bladder, the ends of the ureters (tubes that drain the kidneys), the uterus, ovaries, fallopian tubes, and part of the vagina. If you and your doctor decide that bladder removal or radical cystectomy is your best option, you'll want to be fully informed about what that entails. Chances are you'll wonder what's it really going to be like living without a bladder? First off, you'll be rid of the symptoms from the muscle invasive bladder cancer. No more peeing blood, or worse, passing blood clots, or even worse having those blood clots clog up the urethra, which has resulted in trips to the ER to get the clots irrigated out. If you've had bladder cancer, you've probably discovered that at times the bleeding has been so bad that you've had to be hospitalized after multiple trips to the ER and then OR to resect more tumor and stop the bleeding. Once your bladder is out, the bladder pain will be gone, as well as the horrible symptoms of having the constant urge to pee, being unable to hold it at times, the multiple trips to the bathroom every 30-60 minutes, getting up five to eight times at night to pee and getting no sleep. This is not to say that having your bladder removed is not a life changing experience. It is. But, as bad as it might seem to live without a bladder, living with a bladder that has cancer in it can be an awful experience.

The operation can be done "open" through an incision that starts a few centimeters above the belly button and extends to the pubic bone, or through four to six small incisions using laparoscopes, usually with the aid of the daVinci robot. As more urologists are developing expertise using the robot, most laparoscopic radical cystectomies are being done robotically.

To prepare for the surgery, exercise and increase your caloric intake. If you're a smoker, you are at risk of pulmonary complications, as well as a variety of infections or bleeding. So this is a good time to quit. The day before surgery most surgeons will want you on a clear liquid diet. Some surgeons will also want you to do a bowel prep, but this varies from institution to institution, and even from surgeon to surgeon, so there is no one right way. If it's planned that you will have a urostomy (discussed below) or a catherizable stoma (also discussed below) it's often helpful to meet with a stomal therapist prior to surgery.

There are unique risks and benefits associated with a radical cystectomy. The main benefit to undergoing this major life changing operation is that it may be your best chance of being in the 70% of people with MIBC who are still alive in five years. The other benefit is, as I've already noted, that removing the bladder takes care of debilitating symptoms and bleeding from the cancer itself. Like most major surgeries there is the risk of bleeding, infection, damage to surrounding organs and blood vessels, blood clots, and heart and lung problems related to anesthesia and pre-existing conditions. Depending on how much of the roof of the vagina needs to be removed, vaginal intercourse may be compromised.

The prospect of having all or a part of your vagina removed (vaginectomy) is understandably concerning. If your surgeon can spare any of the vagina, s/he will, and with time and pelvic exercises, you'll be able to resume sexual activity. There may be some dryness and/or loss of sensation, but your physician can prescribe medications to treat that. Fortunately, the vaginal canal is an elastic, muscular structure, so it can be stretched with exercises and even medical dildos designed for that purpose. If you must have it all removed, however, there have been great advances in vaginal reconstruction using skin grafts from your inner thigh. Fortunately, in most cases of cystectomy, a total vaginectomy is unnecessary.

A radical cystectomy is a long operation that can take four to eight hours. The longer the operation, the greater the risk. In addition, there are additional complications related to urinary tract reconstruction.

After the bladder has been removed, there has to be somewhere for the urine to go. In other words, the urinary tract minus the bladder, needs to be reconstructed. This reconstruction is also known as "urinary diversion."

There are two main types of urinary diversion, and several variations of these diversions. For our purposes we'll discuss urinary diversions as "continent" or "incontinent." An example of an incontinent urinary diversion is called an "ileal conduit" or "ileal loop." A type of continent diversion involves what's called a "neobladder" (new bladder). The neobladder can be attached (anastomosed) to your own urethra. The ureters are attached to either the ideal loop or neobladder. Before attaching the ureters to the conduit, the cut ends of the ureters are sent to the pathologist for a frozen section to make sure that there is no cancer in either ureter.

To create an ileal loop, a 12" segment of ilium (small intestine) is separated from the rest of the ilium. The two ends of the ilium are reconnected to reestablish the flow of small bowel contents. One end (the end furthest away from the large intestine) is closed (usually with staples) while the other end is left open. Each ureter (after a negative frozen section) is attached to the loop. The open end of the loop is attached to the skin and becomes the "stoma." A bag (ileostomy bag) is placed over the stoma. Once in place, urine drains from kidneys, down ureters, into the ileal loop, and into the bag.

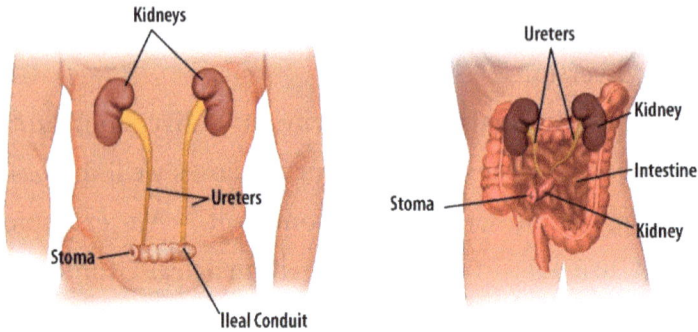

**Urinary diversion, ileal loop (not continent, requires a bag or ileostomy to collect urine, which is worn on the abdomen)**

A continent (no bag needed to collect urine) type of urinary tract reconstruction involves the creation of a neobladder (new bladder). Ileum is again used, only this time a much longer segment is needed to create a pouch. The two ureters are connected to the pouch, and the neobladder is then attached to the urethra. This is called an orthotopic neobladder. Continence depends on the one remaining sphincter, the external sphincter.

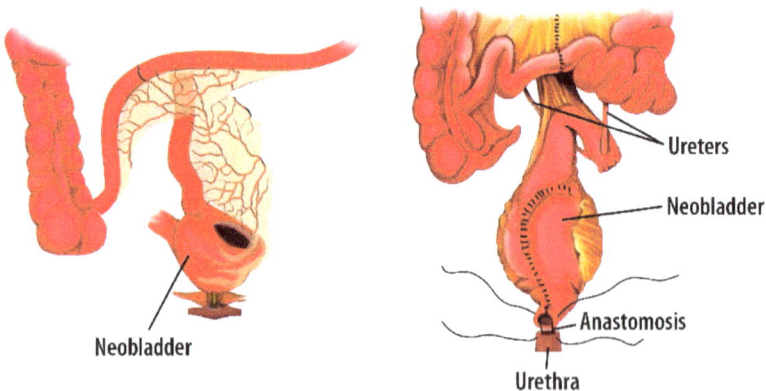

**Orthotopic Neobladder – "new bladder", usually constructed from a segment of small intestine (ileum). The neobladder is attached to the patient's own urethra and is called "orthotopic"**

Because of body habits or internal anatomy, sometimes the neobladder cannot reach the external sphincter so attachment isn't possible. In this case, the pouch can be made "continent" by making a tube about the size of a straw that's formed from the same ileum and is part of the neobladder construction. This tube is attached to the skin in the lower abdomen, or umbilicus. With this type of continent neobladder, the pouch will need to be emptied by inserting a catheter every 2-6 hours to drain the urine.

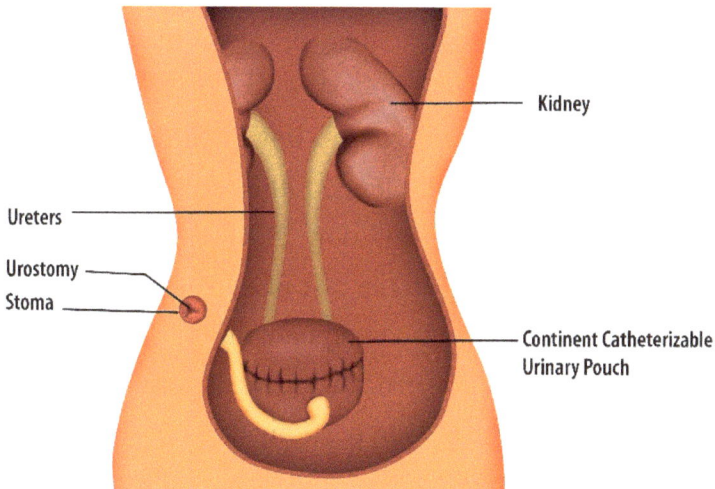

Continent urinary diversion (no bag, but must be catheterized several times a day to empty the pouch of urine)

## Continent Urinary Diversion

The goals of urinary diversion are to preserve renal function and provide adequate urine drainage while at the same time minimizing complications. The benefits of a continent neobladder (either attached to skin, in which case it requires catheterization several times a day or attached to the urethra in which case you would pee in the normal way) are to minimize the impact on your body image, so you will not need to wear a bag to collect urine. The benefits of the ileal loop are that it's simple, quicker, and less likely to have problems. Your urologist will evaluate you to determine whether you're a good candidate for one or the other, based on your age and state of health.

Both types of diversion have potential complications in common. Whenever you make attachments, be it bowel to bowel, ureter to bowel, bowel to urethra, or even bowel to skin, those attachments can scar and become obstructed. The other thing that can happen is that the attachments can leak. Either problem may require another operation to fix.

Whenever you expose urine to bowel, there can be metabolic, acid-base, or electrolyte problems. Either type of diversion can be associated with renal deterioration. Both are associated with an increased risk of infection. In the case of a neobladder, if the pressure gets too high and the urine isn't emptied, the pouch can rupture. Last, sometimes the continence mechanism with each type of continent diversion will not keep a person perfectly dry.

There have been dramatic advances in creation of neobladders, continent diversions, and even the ileal loop as urologists have learned how best to avoid these potential complications. I don't mean to deter you, just to inform you of the possibilities. Not all patients are candidates for neobladders or continent diversions. You will need to rely on the judgement and advice of your urologist.

Aside from having to catheterize and irrigate a cutaneous neobladder, your lifestyle should not be compromised. With an orthotopic neobladder (attached to your own urethra), your "internal new bladder" should be the same as if you have a normal bladder, except for the fact that you may need to periodically irrigate the mucous out to prevent blockage.

I normally don't recommend seeking anecdotal advice from the neighbor or relative who has gone through the same cancer ordeal that you are faced with. In the case of living without your bladder, however, it may be helpful for you to talk to other people who are living without their bladders. Your urologist will know of some of these people who s/he has operated on who are living normal active lives with either diversion. Ask them what it's like, what's involved, and if they would make the same decision if they had to do it again. I promise that this conversation will serve you well, and people who have gone through this are usually happy to help.

## Conclusion

Bladder cancer is not necessarily a death sentence, there's a ray of hope down every avenue, no matter how serious the initial diagnosis is. It may take overcoming obstacles, surgery, chemo, and/or radiation, as all are possible treatments you'll may need. Like other chapters in this book, my aim in this chapter has been to help you discuss your options for therapy with your urologist, oncologist, and radiation oncologist through Shared Decision Making. Hopefully this chapter has provided you with information necessary to have such a conversation with your doctors.

# CHAPTER 7

# Kidney Tumors, Cysts, and Masses

This is a chapter you probably won't be reading unless you or a loved one have, or may have, a tumor or mass in the kidney. Our lives depend on having at least one functioning kidney, yet those of us with healthy kidneys don't think about them all that much. It's only when something goes wrong that we turn our attention to these life supporting organs. Finding a tumor or mass in a kidney is a discovery that gets our attention.

Any tumor or mass in the kidney is cause for concern because it could be cancer. The most common type of kidney cancer is renal cell carcinoma, or RCC. In the United States there will be 73,000 new cases of RCC each year, and 15,000 will die each year. Though anyone can get it, it is more common in men, African Americans, and Native Americans. RCC is an aggressive cancer with a five year survival rate of 35%, which is a discouraging statistic if you receive the diagnosis. Fortunately, there have been significant advances in treatment of renal cell carcinoma of all stages. For localized kidney cancers, those that have not spread outside of the kidney, laparoscopic and robotic assisted laparoscopic removal of either part or all of the kidney have become the norm, which represents a major advance in caring for kidney cancer patients over the past 15 years.

RFA (radiofrequency ablation) and cryoablation (freezing) are good options in certain circumstances, and result in decent cancer control and survival for some patients who may not be able to tolerate a more involved operation. Finally, there have been significant advances with a wide variety of chemotherapeutic agents over the past 15 years. There are ongoing clinical trials that are studying new "targeted" therapy. Survival rates are improving, and should continue to improve, though metastatic kidney cancer is still a very serious condition. So what does it mean for you if you receive the news that a tumor or mass has been detected in one or both kidneys? Let's consider the possibilities.

## Renal Masses

A renal mass is a general term for any abnormal growth in the kidney. Renal masses can be benign or malignant, they can be single or multiple, they may or may not cause pain, they may or may not produce blood in the urine, and they vary in size from a half inch to over ten or more inches. A renal mass can affect all or just a portion of the kidney. Renal masses are often discovered by chance, when doctors are looking for something else, and turn up on an ultrasound, CT scan, or MRI. However a mass is discovered and whatever its state, the first thing your urologist will want to determine is if the mass is solid or cystic.

A cystic mass is one that is filled with fluid. The fluid can be a water-like protein or it may be blood (a "hemorrhagic cyst"). Most renal cysts do not produce symptoms, but depending on the type of renal cyst, it may or may not be malignant. How do you know which type of cyst you have? Your urologist will want you to have diagnostic imaging tests, which will be reviewed by a radiologist and your urologist who will use a series of objective criteria to determine certain characteristics of the cyst. CT scans done for renal lesions, both cystic and solid, are first done prior to the administration of intravenous contrast. After the non-contrast CT, an IV contrast material is injected (which shouldn't cause any pain or discomfort) and the scan is repeated. Renal cysts that have the potential of being malignant will take up the contrast and "light up" or show what's called "contrast enhancement." Those that are benign will not enhance or take up contrast.

Once imaging (usually CT but can also be ultrasound and/or MRI) is completed the results are reviewed. Kidney cysts are classified according to something called the Bosniak classification system, which classifies them as I, II, II-F, III, and IV. A Bosniak I cyst is a simple kidney cyst. These B-I cysts usually do not cause any symptoms unless they become so large that they press upon the surrounding organs, which is rare. B-I cysts are quite common (nearly half of people over 50 have them) and do not need to be treated in any way. A cyst that meets true Bosniak II classification is also benign and does not need treatment. B-II cysts are different on the CT when compared to a B-1 cyst, in that there may be separations within the cyst. These septations look like thin walls that traverse the cyst are usually not calcified. B-II-F cysts are slightly more complicated, however. A B-IIF cyst can have more septa and calcifications, but do not take up contrast or enhance. The "F" stands for "Follow" because even though 75 to 95% of these cysts are benign, some will take on the radiographic appearance of a more ominous cyst later. For that reason, urologists recommend yearly ultrasounds or CT scans to be sure they aren't growing or changing in any way, or in other words, not changing from benign to malignant.

Bosniak III cysts are characterized by multiple septa of varying thickness and can have varying amounts of calcification within them. Fifty percent of B-III cysts are malignant and therefore it's generally recommended that they be removed. A biopsy of B-III cysts is not recommended, because it's easy to miss cancer if present. There are several surgical options for removing the mass including laparoscopic or open surgery. If the location of the mass allows removal of the mass with a "margin" of normal kidney, this is called a "partial nephrectomy." Sometimes, however, a B-III cyst is in the central portion of the kidney and partial removal is not possible because it would either jeopardize the collecting system of the blood vessels that supply or drain blood from the kidney. The bottom line is that no matter the size of the cyst, if it's a B-III, it should be removed.

B-IV cysts are malignant and these, too, need to be removed either by partial or total nephrectomy.

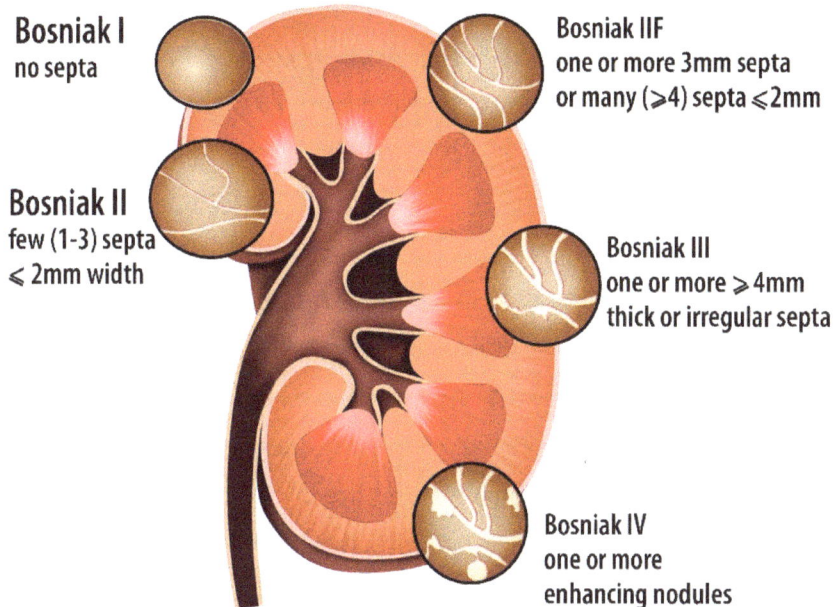

**Bosniak I**
no septa

**Bosniak II**
few (1-3) septa
≤ 2mm width

**Bosniak IIF**
one or more 3mm septa
or many (>4) septa ≤2mm

**Bosniak III**
one or more ≥4mm
thick or irregular septa

**Bosniak IV**
one or more
enhancing nodules

## Bosniak Classification system of kidney cysts

Before we move on to solid renal masses, a few more words about renal cysts. Although rare, cysts can become infected. If this happens, you will usually have flank pain (pain in your upper abdomen, back or sides), fever, and an elevated white blood cell count. A cyst can also rupture, but this is also rare. Cyst rupture is characterized by sudden and sometimes severe flank pain. And a cyst can become so large that is blocks the outflow of urine from the kidney or can press on surrounding organs and cause pain. All three of these conditions are rare, however, so if you are diagnosed with a benign cyst, it's unlikely to cause you any problems.

There is an inherited condition called Adult Polycystic Kidney Disease (APKD). The inheritance pattern can be either autosomal dominant or recessive. If you have APKD, there can be hundreds of cysts in each kidney and the kidneys can be so large that they cause abdominal or flank pain. Sometimes there are so many cysts that they replace the entire functioning tissue of the kidney, which results in renal failure. People with APKD are prone to hypertension. There is an increased association with aneurisms (balloon dilation of blood vessels). Patients with APKD can also have multiple cysts in their liver. Patients with huge kidneys due to APKD can have severe bothersome symptoms (abdominal distention, pain, bloating, nausea and vomiting), simply due to the size of the kidneys. In these cases, it's sometimes necessary to surgically puncture all the cysts to make room for the other abdominal organs. Also, when APKD leads to renal failure, there are times when both non-functioning kidneys are removed before renal transplantation.

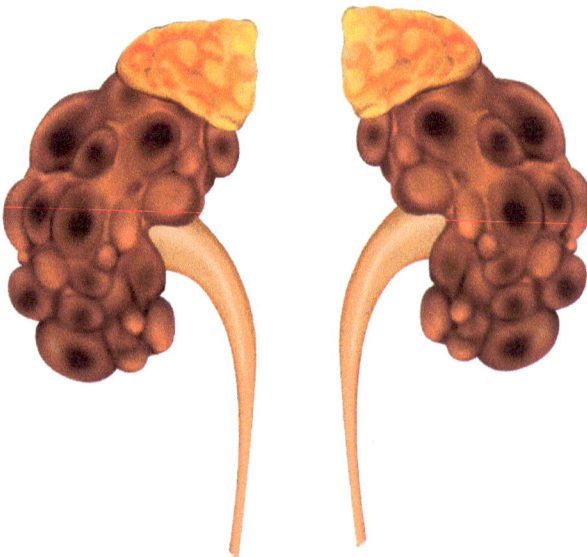

**Adult Polysysistic Kidney Disease**

What if the mass is solid? That's when you're likely wondering, is it cancer? Am I going to die? Well, that depends. The size of the tumor matters. Age matters. Co-morbid conditions matter. What the mass looks like under the microscope matters.

The smaller the solid renal mass, the more likely it is going to be benign. What is small? Well, let's say "small" is less than 0.5 inch or a centimeter. Solid renal tumors that size or less are usually benign. The bigger the mass, however, the more likely it is to be malignant. Yet, not all large renal masses (more than half an inch or 1.0 cm) are malignant. Of those that are malignant, 90% are going to be "renal cell carcinoma" or "adenocarcinoma of the kidney" or "clear cell carcinoma of the kidney." These three names all describe the same cancer, renal cell cancer, what we call RCC or RCCa. As far as your urologist is concerned, all solid renal tumors should be considered RCCa (renal cell cancer) until proven otherwise, even the small ones. So what happens if a solid mass is found?

If you are found to have a solid renal mass, the size and radiologic features (CT/MRI) will point toward it being malignant. Before embarking on treatment, your urologist will want to know if the cancer has spread to other parts of your body. This is called a metastatic work-up. Since kidney cancer is one of the more common cancers to spread to bone, your urologist will order a bone scan and several blood tests. One of the blood tests is called alkaline phosphatase and can be elevated in the presence of bone metastases. Kidney cancer also spreads to lymph nodes in the retroperitoneum, abdomen, chest, and anywhere else in the body where there are lymph nodes. For that reason, a CT scans of the chest is done. You will have already had a CT or MRI of the abdomen and pelvis.

Whether or not to biopsy a solid kidney tumor is a matter of controversy. Some urologists feel that there's no harm in doing a biopsy. But it can be easy to miss RCCa on biopsy, and imaging tests are pretty good in determining whether it's malignant. A biopsy may be indicated if we can't tell whether the mass is benign or malignant based on CT or MRI. My view is that the urologist should ask whether or not a biopsy will affect the treatment they are likely to recommend. For example, a 3.0 cm (golf ball size) solid mass in a 75 year old with multiple medical problems would likely be managed by active surveillance, even if it does enhance on CT/MRI, so the results of a biopsy, whether benign or malignant, would not alter what I'd recommend to my patient, so I would not advise a biopsy. Or say the patient is 50 and has a 5 cm (2 inch) tumor that enhances on CT/MRI and has no fat in it (fat appears as black on imaging, and usually means its benign tumor called an angiomyolipoma). A renal tumor that enhances and has no fat in it is most likely cancer. Removal needs to be done regardless, so why risk a biopsy when it's not going to change what we'd recommend? Or consider my friend's 86 year old mother, who was suffering from dementia when a solid mass was found in her right kidney. She most likely had a malignancy. However, because of her age and other medical problems, she would not benefit from having surgery, so even if the biopsy proved that it was malignant, we would not recommend that it be removed. If the patient were younger, however, and we couldn't tell by imaging if the mass was benign or malignant, a biopsy could be in order because if it showed benign tissue, the patient could avoid having unnecessary surgery.

A biopsy of a renal mass should be considered when the results will change what you would do about it. There are cases when the radiologist and urologist will be unable to tell if the mass is malignant or benign. There are other solid masses of the kidney that are not benign, but they aren't primary kidney tumors, which means they didn't originate in the kidney. Examples of non-renal cancers of the kidney are lymphomas or metastatic lesions from a non-renal source, like breast or GI cancers, or melanoma. In the case of lymphoma, chemotherapy, not surgery, is usually the first and best treatment option. Certain infectious processes can also look like renal masses, and these problems are usually treated with antibiotics. Some infectious renal masses become abscesses and may require surgical drainage.

## Stage and Grade

Let's assume you are anxiously awaiting the results of your testing when your urologist breaks the bad news: you have kidney cancer. What's next? Your treatment will depend upon the stage and grade of your cancer. How is renal cancer stage and grade determined, and why is it important? Stage refers to the size and extent of the cancer, and grade refers to what the cancer looks like under the microscope—the appearance of the cells and the architecture of how the cells are arranged. The more abnormal the individual cells appear and the more abnormal the architecture, the higher the grade.

The staging system most often used for most cancers including kidney and bladder cancer worldwide is the **TNM** system. The "T" stands for tumor and refers to the size of the mass, how much of the organ (in this case the kidney) the tumor occupies, whether it has grown into critical structures within the kidney, if it's grown beyond the boundary of the outer kidney capsule into the surrounding fat, and if it had grown into surrounding organs. A number 1-4 is assigned to the T stage. The lower the number, the better.

The spread to lymph nodes is signified by "N." Your urologist will want to know if the cancer has spread to nearby lymph nodes or distant lymph nodes. The N "number" varies according to which lymph nodes are positive (adjacent to the kidney, or distant), how many nodes appear positive, and the size of the positive nodes. If surgery hasn't been done yet, the N number is assessed by imaging (CT, MRI, or PET). If nodes are removed at the same time the kidney cancer is removed, and they have cancer in them, the N number is based on what they find.

The "M" stands for metastasis. Renal cell carcinoma spreads to other parts of the body by getting into the blood or lymphatic vessels. RCC has an affinity for spreading to bone and lung, and rarely to brain, liver, adrenal gland, and pancreas. If you have metastatic disease, your urologist, a radiation oncologist, and medical oncologist will work together to determine the best course of treatment. There are circumstances in which a person may have metastatic disease and depending on the number and location of the metastasis, all three treatment modalities (radiation, chemo, and surgery) may be recommended. There are other circumstances in which surgery will be of no benefit, and it would be best to treat you with chemo alone.

The TNM assigned to each kidney cancer is determined before surgery. This is the "clinical" stage and is based on physical exam, possible biopsies (tumor, lymph nodes, bone), and imaging tests (CT, MRI, bone and PET scans). If surgery is done, the "pathologic" stage is determined by examining tissue (the tumor itself, possibly the entire kidney with the tumor in it if the whole thing is removed, and possibly lymph nodes if a node dissection is done). This cancer staging may be complex and confusing so if you have any questions about your TNM stage, please ask your doctor to explain it to you in a way you understand. Along with tumor grade, the stage is important in what treatment options are best for your particular situation.

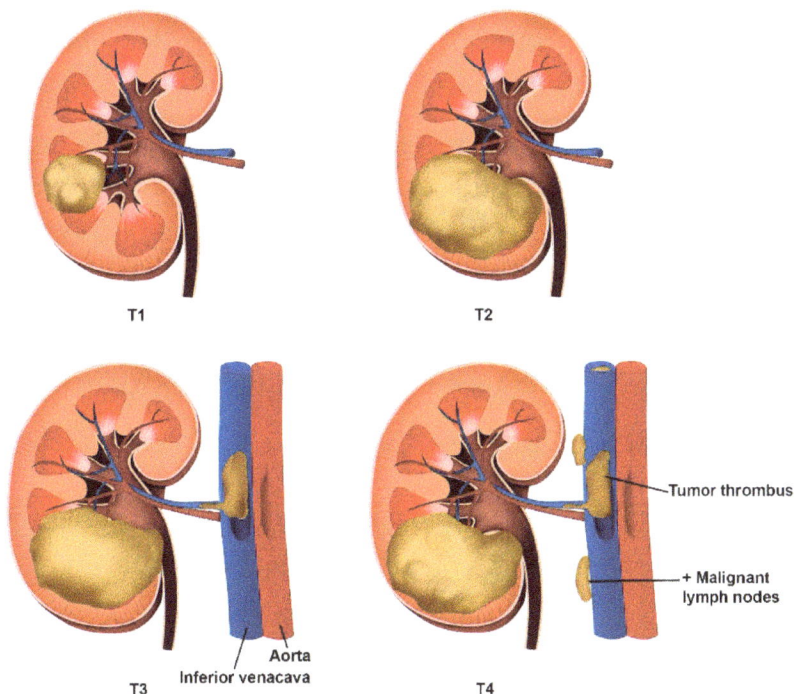

T1

T2

Tumor thrombus

+ Malignant lymph nodes

Aorta
Inferior venacava

T3

T4

## Stages of kidney cancer – renal cell carcinoma

In addition to stage and grade, your age, general health status, and any existing co-morbidities, also play a role in deciding which treatment options are best. For cancers confined to the kidney (T1 and T2), laparoscopic and robotic assisted laparoscopic removal of either part or all of the kidney have become the norm. Radiofrequency ablation (RFA) and cryoablation (freezing) are good options in certain circumstances, and result in decent cancer control and survival for some patients who may not be able to tolerate a more involved operation.

There have also been significant advances with a wide variety of chemotherapeutic agents over the past 15 years. There are ongoing clinical trials that are studying new "targeted" therapy. Survival rates are improving, and should continue to improve, though metastatic kidney cancer is still a very serious condition. If you are unfortunate to have Stage IV metastatic renal cell carcinoma, you will best be served by an oncologist who is familiar with the variety of newer chemotherapy strategies, and the ongoing clinical trials that employ these new drugs.

## Conclusion

In summary, if you are seeing a urologist for a kidney tumor, you'll want to know if it's cystic or solid, benign or malignant. If your urologist can't tell, you'll want to be aware of how you can find out using various imaging techniques, and possibly having the mass biopsied. If your urologist says it's most likely benign, you'll want to know what you need to do to follow it to be sure it stays benign, that is, will it grow or change into something that's malignant? Some benign kidney tumors (angiomyolipoma, for example), can grow quite large. As these benign tumors increase in size (bigger than a plum or 4.5 cm) they are more likely to bleed, which can be catastrophic.

If the mass is malignant, you'll also want to participate in a Shared Decision Making discussion with your urologist and learn about the various options for treatment, the risks and potential benefits of each treatment option, and the differences in the 5, 10, and 15 year survival. Don't hesitate to write your questions down. "If I have just the part of the kidney with the tumor in it removed, or removal just the tumor, as opposed to removing all the kidney and tumor, is there a difference in survival?" "What are the potential complications of a robotic assisted lap nephrectomy (kidney removal using laparoscopes and the robot)? How are those complications different from an open nephrectomy? What's the difference in how many days I'll be in the hospital? What's the difference in recovery time, when will I be able to play pickleball again?" "Would I benefit from having chemo before you take my kidney tumor out?" "Do I need to see an oncologist? Radiation oncologist?" "What would happen if I don't have surgery?" And more.

Yes, there are lots of questions. I'll frequently get a call from a friend, relative, or friend of a friend saying "They say I have a kidney tumor and that it might be cancer. What should I ask the urologist?" I hope that this chapter will help answer your questions. Ideally your urologist will have the time to go through all your options so that you and they can arrive at the best decision.

# CHAPTER 8

# Emergencies and Trauma

If you are unlucky enough to have experienced trauma to the genitourinary system, you were likely seen in the emergency room or urgent care. Isolated urologic trauma is rare. Most urologic trauma also involves other organ systems. For example, when there is a significant abdominal injury, ten percent of those injuries involve urologic organs. And fractured lower ribs or a fractured pelvis should put the provider on alert for a possible urologic injury.

Trauma can be categorized as blunt force (such as from motor vehicle accident, a fall, a sports injury like a hard tackle in football, or being hit by a car while walking or riding a bike) or penetrating (gunshot wounds, stabbings, or impalement).

All organs of the GU system are at risk from such injuries, from the top of the kidney to the end of the urethra. Any injury to the lower abdomen or pelvis can injure the bladder, urethra, reproductive organs, and genitalia. An injury to the lower chest (including fractured ribs) or upper abdomen will usually prompt rapid evaluation in the ER with a CT scan. One sign that ER doctors look for is blood in the urine, either microscopic or blood that can be seen with the naked eye. This may be a sign of an injury to the kidney. Kidney injuries can be mild or severe. Kidney injuries are graded 1 (mild or a contusion, like a kidney bruise) to 4 (severe, which is a shattered kidney or injury to one of the blood vessels going to or from the kidney). Some mild kidney injuries are observed, knowing that they will heal on their own, while other more severe injuries require surgery, which sometimes involves removing the kidney.

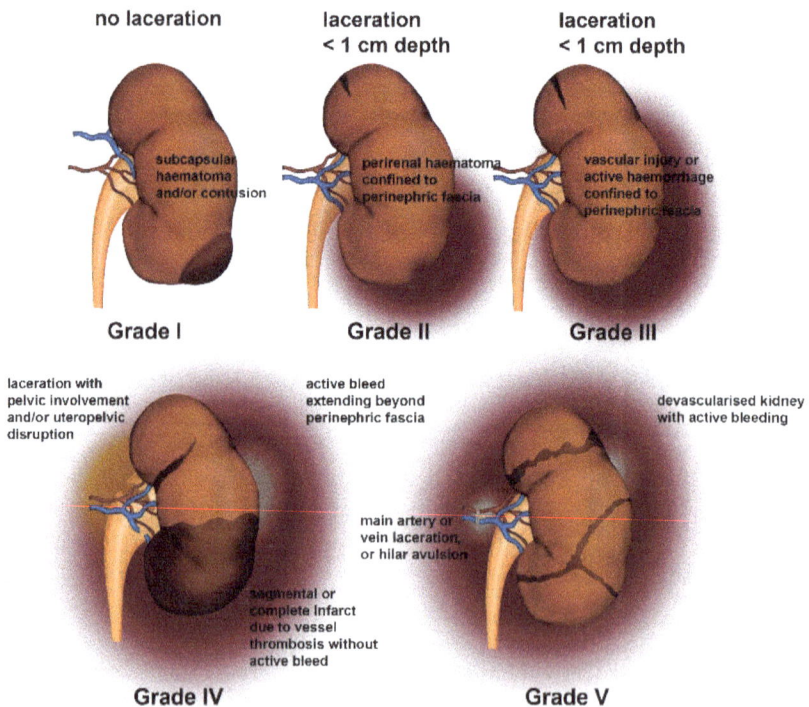

no laceration

laceration < 1 cm depth

laceration < 1 cm depth

subcapsular haematoma and/or contusion

perirenal haematoma confined to perinephric fascia

vascular injury or active haemorrhage confined to perinephric fascia

Grade I

Grade II

Grade III

laceration with pelvic involvement and/or uteropelvic disruption

active bleed extending beyond perinephric fascia

devascularised kidney with active bleeding

main artery or vein laceration, or hilar avulsion

segmental or complete infarct due to vessel thrombosis without active bleed

Grade IV

Grade V

**5 grades of blunt renal trauma**

Injuries to the lower abdomen and pelvis can result in either a bladder injury, urethral injury, or both. Again, the CT scan is useful in determining if there is an injury to the bladder and/or urethra. Like the kidney, some of these injuries can be observed, while others will require surgery.

## Catheters

Catheters are necessary and helpful, but they can at times cause problems. Generally speaking, catheters are soft hollow tubes that are used to drain fluid from the body. Catheters are used by a variety of medical specialists, including urologists. In addition to being used to drain fluid (like urine), they can also be placed in spaces to measure certain physiologic metrics (like pressure in a chamber of the heart), or to inject substances for treating certain conditions (like when you want to block blood flow to a part of a certain organ that is bleeding, the interventional radiologist can embolize the blood vessel by placing a coil through a catheter).

Urinary catheters are like double-edged swords. On the one hand, they are necessary and useful in draining urine from places where urine for whatever reason won't drain. On the other hand, aside from being uncomfortable, when a catheter is displaced or removed before its time, or if it gets obstructed or breaks, it can cause significant problems.

Urologists are experts at urinary catheters. Catheters put into the bladder are called Foley catheters, named after American urologist Frederic Foley, who invented a self-retaining catheter in 1929. Foley developed a catheter with a balloon toward the bladder end of the catheter that could be filled with water through a separate port. It might surprise you to learn that Foley wasn't the first to invent a flexible catheter—Benjamin Franklin invented the first flexible catheter (though without the balloon) in 1752 when he was looking for a way to help his brother James who suffered from bladder and kidney stones. Apparently there wasn't much Ben Franklin didn't succeed at!

Catheters have proven to be remarkable, yet simple, devices for resolving all sorts of issues, and for us urologists, essential to our daily work. Urologists are frequently called about catheter issues. Emergency calls come from all sorts of places—emergency rooms, ICUs, med-surg wards, outpatient offices, nursing homes, just about anywhere someone has a catheter, a misadventure can occur.

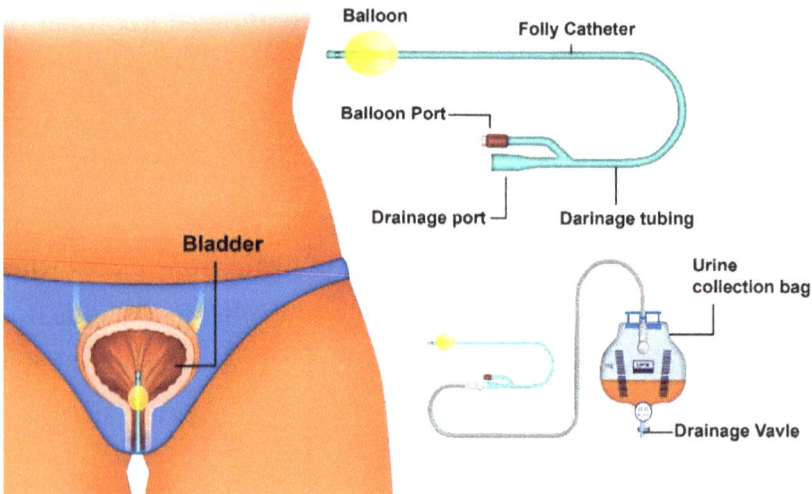

**Urinary Foley Catheter**

## Blunt and Penetrating Injuries

Blunt and penetrating injuries are relatively rare in women but they do occur, and when they do they can affect any part of the urinary tract from the top of the kidney to the tip of the urethra. Foreign bodies such as a broken off piece of a catheter can also find a home in the urinary tract and cause bleeding, infection, or obstruction. I've had to remove foreign bodies from female bladders that were intended for the vagina and somehow the wrong orifice (urethra) was entered.

## Intra-Operative Injuries

Gynecologists and urologists operate in the same territory. Some surgeries, like C-sections or hysterectomies, can be difficult due to unusual anatomy or scar tissue from previous surgery or infection. Rarely, the bladder or one of the ureters will be injured during these difficult cases. When that happens, urologists are called in to help repair the injury. If the ureter is inadvertently cut or occluded, part of the repair process may involve a stent or a drainage tube (nephrostomy tube) in the kidney in order for the repair to heal.

## Conclusion

Injuries and emergencies involving the urinary tract are unexpected. If and when they do happen, rest assured that the urologist called to your emergent situation is well trained to do the right thing to fix the injury, with the goal in mind to preserve kidney, bladder, and ureter function, and to make you whole and healthy again.

# CONCLUSION

I wrote this book in an effort to help patients make better decisions about their urinary healthcare, to have a better sense of their health concerns, and to have informed, shared decision making discussions with their urologists.

When I was actively practicing urology at Kaiser Permanente in Portland, where I had practiced for 31 years, I was bothered by not having enough time to counsel my patients. This was true for all patients, including those with blood in their urine, kidney stones, people who couldn't pee, or peed too much. All were worried, and all had questions—but there wasn't enough time to answer their questions and concerns in the limited time available.

Women with newly diagnosed cancer deserved better. I had either phoned them with the cancer diagnosis, or they were coming in to get the bad news. Yet I had only 15 minutes for a discussion of the results and what comes next. When done properly, a shared decision making conversation about a new diagnosis of cancer takes at least an hour. That discussion never happened to my or my patient's satisfaction. Instead, they would leave the office confused, depressed, and anxious. Some would go on the internet and Google "treatment of bladder cancer" or "kidney cancer," as well as "life expectancy," "survival rate" and other dire word strings reflecting their understandable fears. Some would talk to relatives or neighbors who had been through cancer treatment. Whatever they did, they would inevitably return a week or two later full of misinformation, more confusion, and more anxiety.

When I retired in 2014, I needed something to do. I decided to write down all the information I wanted my patients (and their families) to know when they came to me with bladder or renal cancer, infections, urinary problems, or any of a number of things that people commonly suffer but know little about. And I know they want answers because the questions didn't stop with my retirement. To this day I still get a lot of questions, sometimes three or four a week. A lot of these questions are raised on the golf course, or from friends, or friends of friends, often when my mind is far from the topic of urology as I focus on my next shot.

I started playing semi-serious competitive golf. It seemed that every time I got paired with a new partner, after finding out I was a urologist, questions inevitably followed. "I've had lots of stones, lots of surgery and procedures for my stones, is there anything I can do to stop them?" Or "my wife had bladder cancer and they took her bladder out a couple of years ago. Did she really have to go through all that?" or "My wife is miserable, she has to go to the bathroom every 30 minutes, it's driving us nuts. Shouldn't she see a urologist?"

In 2015 I started volunteering for the M.A.V.E.N. project (Medical Advice Volunteer Expert Network https://www.mavenproject.org/) as a clinical consultant. The MAVEN project provides health consultation to over 200 clinics for the uninsured in 19 states. None of these clinics have specialists, they are all staffed by primary care providers (generalists, internists, family practitioners, nurse practitioners, and physician assistants). Whenever these PCPs require specialty consultation for their patients, they submit an electronic consult. Almost every specialty you can imagine is represented by a volunteer physician in that specialty. As I started responding to these requests for help with urology, I realized that it wasn't just those on the golf course who had questions—the PCPs were thirsting for information and guidance, and so were their uninsured patients.

So, I flipped open my laptop and started writing about the common urologic conditions that brought men and women to my office, the stuff I was asked about both on the golf course and by the MAVEN PCPs. When I was done, if someone on the golf course asked me a question, I'd send them the relevant chapter. When a MAVEN PCP working in a free clinic wanted a consult on a kidney tumor, I'd send the chapter on renal masses. Soon, the feedback I received made it clear that I needed a better way to disseminate this information to those who had questions. And that brings me to you.

This book is for you. I'm assuming you are a non-medical person with a urologic problem, or someone you care about has a urologic issue. You may be one of the women I play golf with who has seen blood in your urine, or you may have been told there's a mass in your kidney, or  a tumor in your bladder. Whatever your issue, I know you're concerned, and I know you want—and need—more information.

Whatever inspired you to open this book, however, it is not meant to substitute for a conversation between you and your doctor. I've written these chapters to supplement the conversation most doctors do not have half the time to provide you – time you need, and time that our modern healthcare system has made nearly impossible for them to provide. The material I've gone over in this book is meant to help you wade through the millions of "hits" you will get when you Google your problem whether, "how do I get rid of a kidney stone" or "what does it mean if there's blood in my urine?" If anything, *this book will save you and your doctor time.*

I have also tried to be frank without alarming you, as well as evidence based. Personal bias enters into every doctor's decision—one might favor one way of taking care of a problem over another, or one might think that one drug is superior to another, or that one way of taking a kidney stone out is superior to an alternative. This physician bias comes into play frequently. Sometimes treatments are equal, but the risks are different. Sometimes one treatment will be better than an alternative but has different and potentially more dangerous risks. And your values, needs, and preferences are different from the next patient's. I've tried taking all these factors into consideration in the discussions of your urinary health concerns.

Decisions you make about your urologic health are not easy. There's a lot to know, and a lot to consider. Most times decisions are best when patients fully understand their issue, what the possible options are for addressing the problem, and the potential risks and benefits of the potential treatments. My hope is that this book will help you and your doctor share in making the best decision for you and for the people you love.

# APPENDIX I

# Glossary

**adenocarcinoma** - malignant cancer that originates from glandular tissue

**adjuvant, neo-adjuvant chemotherapy** - additional therapy added to another cancer treatment, for example, radiation after surgery. Neo-adjuvant therapy is additional therapy that is given before another therapy, for example, chemotherapy before surgery.

**adrenal glands** - triangular shaped glands about 1" high and 3" long composed of an inner (medulla) and outer (cortex) layer. The medulla makes adrenaline and noradrenaline, while the cortex makes other hormones that control  blood pressure, part of the immune system, and other metabolic processes. You normally have two, one on top of each kidney.

**adrenaline (noradrenaline)** - stress hormones (same as epinephrine and norepinephrine) produced by adrenal glands. These hormones are secreted during stress ("flight or fight" response), and play a role in heart rate, breathing rate, sugar and carbohydrate metabolism, and muscle function.

**adult polycystic kidney disease (APKD)** - An inherited genetic (autosomal dominant) disease affecting 1 in 1000 people characterized by multiple cysts in both kidneys. Symptoms usually show up in people in their 30s and 40s.

**alpha blocker** - typically these are drugs that lower blood pressure. Tamsulosin (Flomax) is a specific type of alpha blocker that does not lower blood pressure primarily, but rather relaxes smooth muscle of urinary tract organs (ureters, bladder neck, prostate). The main use of alpha blockers in urology is to aid in urination, bladder emptying, and relaxing the ureter to aid in stone passage.

**anastomosis** - attachment between two structures, such as bladder to urethra, ureter to ureter, blood vessels, renal pelvis to ureter, segments of intestine to intestine, ureter to intestine, and more.

**anatrophic nephrolithotomy** - an open procedure through a flank incision for very large kidney stones in which the solid tissue of the kidney is bivalved to get the stone out. This procedure has been rarely done since 1985

**angiomyolipoma of the kidney**- a solid benign mass of the kidney made up of fat, blood vessels and muscle. Diagnosis is often made by CT scan that shows fat in the mass. AMLs can grow and although benign, if > 5.0 can cause life threatening bleeding. Usually asymptomatic, but when large can be painful.

**anterior repair** – a procedure done in women for bladder prolapse. May involve placement of "mesh" and done at the same time as a "pubovaginal sling".

**arteriole** - a small arterial blood vessel branch off an artery before draining into a capillary.

**artery** - a blood vessel that carries blood and oxygen from the heart to tissues and organs in the body.

**asymptomatic** - without symptoms.

**atrophy** – when an organ or tissue wastes away or shrinks as a result of being deprived of oxygen, blood, and nutrients.

**bacteria** - single cell organisms seen only under the microscope, lacking a nucleus, and present in the large intestine where they do more good than harm. There are many different types and shapes and present in many environments including water, soil, and organic matter.

**benign** - not cancer, not harmful.

**BUN** - blood urea nitrogen. Protein is broken down in the liver. Urea is a waste product of this process. The kidneys filter the blood and add urea and nitrogen to urine. Urea nitrogen levels rise in the blood when the kidneys aren't working properly and in cases of dehydration, heart failure, high protein diet, and certain medication.

**bacteriuria** - bacteria in the urine, sometimes associated with infection and inflammation, other times without infection.

**bilirubin** - a blood test that measures a byproduct of hemoglobin break down in the liver.

**CBC** - a blood test that stands for complete blood count that measures the number of red blood cells, white bloods cells, and platelets.

**calcium oxalate** - crystals that are made from a salt of calcium and oxalate and form the most common urinary tract stone.

**calculus** - a stone formed from mineral salts and organic material found in the kidney, ureter, bladder, prostate, urethra (can also form in the gall bladder, pancreas, ducts draining both liver and pancreas).

**cancer** - a malignant growth or tumor that results from uncontrolled growth of abnormal cells, glands, and tissue.

**carcinoma in situ (CIS)** - growth of cancer cells in the tissue layer of origin seen under the microscope. For our purposes, the lining of the bladder, ureters, prostatic urethra, or hollow lining of the kidney collecting system. Can be seen in other organ systems in which the term takes on different meaning (breast, lung, skin, for example).

**checkpoint inhibitor chemotherapy** - your immune system normally has "checkpoints" that prevent an over response to normal tissues and organs in your body. The checkpoints also prevent your immune system from responding to cancer and tumors. These are drugs that block or inhibit the "checkpoints" and allow your immune system to eradicate the tumor or cancer cells. These drugs have been effective in treating cancers like melanoma and some lung cancers. Over the past 10 years ongoing clinical trials are looking at treating a variety of urological cancers, particularly renal cell carcinoma and bladder cancer.

**chemo/chemotherapy** - a variety of drugs that all have different mechanisms of action designed to treat cancer. The main type of chemo is "cytotoxic," which means "kills cells."

**citrate** - a salt of citric acid which inhibits calcium stone formation. An antioxidant, citrate is found in a variety of fruits and vegetable (lemons, grapefruit, avocado, prunes, and more).

**creatinine** - a chemical that can be measured in blood and urine. Creatinine is a byproduct of the chemical process of energy production by muscles. Healthy kidneys filter blood and add creatinine to urine, which is excreted (peed out) as a waste product. When kidneys are not working properly or in the case of severe dehydration, creatinine levels to rise in the blood.

**cryoablation** - a process of freezing tissue or tumors to super cold temperatures that results in cellular death. Used in urology for treatment of prostate and kidney tumors.

**CT scan** - computerized tomography commonly called a "cat scan." Uses images of multiple x-rays taken in a variety of directions, then fed into a computer that reconstructs the image to resemble a facsimile of tissue, organs, and bones of your body.

**CT urogram** - computerized tomography (CT) to evaluate the urinary tract consisting of kidneys, ureters, bladder, and prostate (men). During the urogram phase of the study, x-ray dye or contrast is injected in a vein in the arm or hand and is then taken up by the kidneys (or kidney tumor) and excreted into the urinary tract.

**cyst** - a fluid contained by a smooth, thin walled sac-like structure.

**cystectomy, simple** - removal of the urinary bladder (simple).

**cystectomy, radical** - removal of the urinary bladder and prostate in a man; removal of the urinary bladder and roof of the vagina, urethra, and the uterus in a female.

**cystinuria** - cystine is an amino acid similar to lysine, ornithine, arginine. Cystinuria is an inherited disorder in which large amount of cystine and cystine crystals are in the urine and form stones.

**cystoscopy** - a procedure done with a flexible fiberoptic scope to enable the urologist to look at the inside of the urethra, bladder, and prostate.

**cystitis** - infection or inflammation (or both) of the bladder.

**cystometrogram** - a procedure done with a catheter in the bladder that measures pressure in the bladder as the bladder fills with saline.

**double J stent (JJ stent)** - a thin flexible plastic hollow tube that resides in the ureter with one "J" or curl in the hollow part of the kidney, and the other J in the bladder. The stent allows drainage of urine from kidney to bladder in order to bypass obstruction from stones, tumor, or scar tissue.

**dihydrotestosterone (DHT)** - a male hormone that is a byproduct of testosterone metabolism. Testosterone is converted to dihydrotesterone by an enzyme called 5 alpha reductase. This conversion is blocked by drugs called 5 alpha reductase inhibitors (Proscar/finasteride, Avodart/dutersteride).

**diverticulum** - a sac or a tube that forms because of a weakness in the wall of a hollow organ or occurs because of increased pressure in that organ. Can also be congenital. Diverticulum can be found in the kidney, ureter, or bladder, and can vary in size from tiny (1/4 inch) to large (tennis ball).

**embolization** – a procedure to stop the flow of blood using tiny coils, beads, or sponges to therapeutically stop the flow of blood to an organ.

**endoscope** - a fiber optic instrument that is used to examine the inside of a body cavity.

**endourology** - the specialized area of urology that employs minimally invasive techniques using endoscopes to treat a variety of problems, particularly urinary tract stones.

**ESWL** - extracorporeal (outside the body) shockwave lithotripsy (break up stones), a non-invasive procedure that uses shockwaves focused using x-rays or ultrasound to break up stones in the urinary tract (has also been used in the biliary tract draining the liver, and the pancreas).

**erythropoietin** - a hormone made in the kidney that stimulates production of red blood cells in bone marrow.

**external sphincter** - the skeletal muscle of the pelvic floor through which the urethra passes. You open and close the external sphincter if you stop and start your urinary stream. You can strengthen the external sphincter doing Kegel's exercises. The external sphincter is the remaining sphincter that maintains continence after the prostate is removed.

**fluoroscopy** - a continuous x-ray beam like an x-ray "video."

**fungus** - a microorganism more complicated than bacteria or viruses. Certain fungi are pathogenic, meaning they can cause disease. examples are candida (yeast), and coccidioimycosis (Valley Fever).

**GI** - gastrointestinal. The GI tract includes the esophagus, stomach, small intestine, large intestine, rectum, liver, biliary system, and pancreas.

**glans penis/clitoris** - the head of the penis. the female equivalent is the clitoris.

**glucose** - a simple sugar made of 6 carbon atoms that is an important energy source for many organisms.

**hematuria, microscopic** - blood in urine that can be seen only under the microscope.

**hematuria, gross** - blood in urine that can be seen with the naked eye and ranging from light pink to dark red with blood clots

**hemorrhagic cyst** - a cyst in the kidney that has blood in it. A hemorrhagic cyst has characteristic ultrasound, CT, and MRI appearance.

**hydrocele** - a fluid (serum) filled sac in the scrotum that contains the testicle and epididymis. In an infant, a hydrocele is always associated with a hernia.

**ileus** - small or large bowel paralysis in response to abdominal or retroperitoneal pain, toxins, or surgery.

**ileal conduit/ileal loop** - a segment of small intestine (usually ilium) to which are attached the ureters draining urine from the kidneys. One end is closed, and the other end fixed to the skin, which is called a stoma of ileostomy.

**infection** - a state in which a bug (usually bacteria or virus) causes illness in a host.

**inflammation** - your body's immune response to infection or injury, can be chronic or acute.

**internal sphincter** - one of three valves in men that are responsible for continence (the prostate and external sphincter are the other two) and in women it's one of two valves (the external sphincter being the 2nd). It is located at the junction of the bladder and prostate in men, and bladder and urethra in women. It is an involuntary sphincter made of smooth (as opposed to skeletal) muscle.

**intra-vesical therapy** - Drugs (chemotherapy, immunotherapy, other) that are instilled into the bladder, typically for treating bladder cancer and interstitial cystitis.

**IVP/IU** - Intravenous pyelogram/intravenous urogram, a procedure more of historical interest because it's been replaced by CTU, rarely done anymore, wherein dye is injected into a vein followed by x-tomography of the kidneys, then sequential x-rays of the bladder.

**ketones** - a breakdown product of fat metabolism. When you are fasting and your body has exhausted its supply of carbohydrates (sugars, glucose, etc.) for energy, the liver will breakdown fat for energy. The by products are ketones, which causes them to show up in the urine. Small amounts of ketones on urine analysis are normal.

**leukocyte** - A white blood cell made by bone marrow important in fighting infection and other ailments. Part of the immune and inflammatory response to a variety of problems.

**laparoscope** - a thin instrument with a camera and a light on the end. The camera displays an image on a video monitor (TV screen). A "working channel" is part of the scope and allows surgeons to pass instruments that allow surgeons to perform a variety of tasks.

**laparoscopic surgery** - a form of "minimally invasive" (MIP) abdominal and/or retroperitoneal surgery done using laparoscopes through one-inch incisions.

**lithotripsy** - any procedure that results in "breaking up stones."

**lumen** - a tube, tubular organ, channel, or cavity.

**malignant** - refers to cancer, meaning the cells grow in an uncontrolled way. The cells have a typical appearance under the microscope. Tumors made up of malignant cells are more prone to grow rapidly and spread to other parts of the body.

**margin positive disease** - after a tumor specimen is removed the outer edges are marked with a special ink. The pathologist then examines tissue from the specimen in a systematic way. If the cancer cells abut the inked margin then there is margin positive disease.

**metastatic** - cancer that has spread via blood or lymph to other parts or organs of the body. For many urologic cancers, that means lymph nodes and bones, but does not exclude other organs (liver, lung, brain, other).

**metastatic workup** - a series of tests that are done to see if cancer has spread, typically to include a bone scan, CT or MRI scans of chest and abdomen (and sometimes head), PET scans, and PSMA scans.

**MIBC** - muscle invasive bladder cancer. Bladder cancer (usually transitional cell cancer) that invades muscle.

**minimally invasive procedure (MIP)** - surgery or other procedures done with limited amount of cutting, or through very small incisions. Examples include robotic laparoscopic surgery, cryotherapy, and several outpatient procedures for BPH. Hopeful benefits are less pain, fewer complications, quicker recovery time, less scarring, less stress on the immune system, smaller or no incision (ESWL).

**mucosa** - the lining layer of any hollow organ. Urinary bladder, ureter, kidney, stomach, intestine (large and small), all have a mucosal lining layer. The glands of this lining layer make mucous.

**neoadjuvant therapy** - for cancer, therapy done before the main therapy, such as chemotherapy done before surgery, in order to shrink the tumor or make it more susceptible to treatment (e.g., hormone ablative neoadjuvant therapy before radiation for prostate cancer).

**neobladder** - a "new" or replacement urinary bladder constructed out of intestine. A form of urinary diversion. When the pouch (neobladder) is attached to the urethra, near normal urination may resume. This is called "orthotopic." When the pouch is attached to the abdominal skin and a bag to collect urine is not necessary, it's called a "continent neobladder."

**nephron** - one of the millions of microscopic units of the kidney that filters blood, removes wastes, regulates electrolytes and other bodily chemicals, and then adds to what is not needed water to make urine.

**nephrostomy tube** - or "neph tube" is a soft flexible tube ranging in size from 1/4" to 1/2" (in adults) that directly drains urine from the internal hollow part of the kidney through a small incision, usually in the back.

**neurotransmitter** - chemical made by nerve cells that sends a message to other nerve cells, muscle cells, and organs. The specific message results in a specific effect. For example, a neurotransmitter is sent via nerves to the penis that results in an erection.

**NMIBC** - non-muscle invasive bladder cancer (see MIBC).

**nocturia** - urination during the night.

**NSAID** - non-steroidal anti-inflammatory, examples are ibuprofen, Advil, Motrin, aspirin.

**OAB** - overactive bladder.

**oncologist** - a doctor (MD or DO) who specializes in the diagnosis and treatment of cancer.

**orthotropic neobladder** - an internal reservoir for urine that replaces the urinary bladder. It is normally constructed from small intestine. Orthotropic means that it is attached to the urethra so that the patient urinates in the usual way.

**osteoporosis** - weak, fragile, brittle bones that results from loss of bone tissue, caused by hormone changes like androgen deprivation therapy, vitamin D and/or calcium deficiency.

**oxalate** - a salt of oxalic acid the occurs in a variety of plants, vegetables, nuts, and other edible food. In urine when combined with calcium forms calcium oxalate stones.

**partial nephrectomy** - a surgery in which a part of the kidney that contains a tumor or disease is removed.

**percutaneous nephrostolithotmy (PERC or PNL)** - a surgical procedure done through a small incision in the back in which a tube is passed into the kidney to remove stones. Usually reserved for larger stones, obstructions downstream from the kidney, or when other less invasive methods are not likely to succeed.

**perineum** - the area of the body between the scrotum and anus in men, and the vagina and anus in women.

**peritoneal cavity** - the cavity in the abdomen that contains the stomach, liver, small intestines, spleen, etc. contained by a membrane called the peritoneum.

**pH** - the acid base status of fluids in the body - blood, urine, intestinal contents, measured on a scale of 1 (very acid) to 14 (very base), where a pH of 7 is neutral. Normal pH for blood is 7.4. Normal urine pH ranges from 4.5 to 8.

**placebo** - a pill, treatment, or procedure that has no physiologic effect, such as a sugar pill or water, or a fake operation. Used as a "control" when evaluating new drugs or procedures.

**posterior repair** - a procedure done on the floor of the vagina to fix prolapse of the rectum frequently done in conjunction with a mid-urethral sling.

**post void residual (PVR)** - the amount of urine in the bladder after urination measured by ultrasound or catheterization.

**PCP** - primary care provider (Family Practice MD, Internist, Physician Assistant, Nurse Practitioner, Pediatrician).

**psychogenic impotence** - Inability to obtain or maintain an erection when all vascular,

**pyelonephritis** - inflammation of the kidney usually from a bacterial infection that presents as flank pain, and usually fever, and sweats, and sometimes nausea and vomiting.

**pyelolithotomy** - an operation in which a stone is removed from the renal pelvis, the hollow internal part of the kidney that stores and then transports urine from the kidney to the ureter.

**radiation oncologist** - an MD or DO who specializes in treating cancers using radiation therapy.

**radiation therapy** - treatment of disease, particularly cancer, using x-rays and a variety of other forms of radiation.

**re-canalization** - situations in which a bodily tube or channel like the vas deferens is blocked or obstructed and a new channel is created to restore flow in the tube.

**renal cell carcinoma** (RCC, same as adenocarcinoma of the kidney, and clear cell carcinoma) - most common type of kidney cancer that is the result of uncontrolled glandular tissue of the kidney producing a solid tumor.

**renal colic** - severe flank pain which is the is the result of blockage along the course of the ureter from where it joins the kidney down to the bladder. Causes of obstruction include stones, scars, congenital narrowing of the ureter (UPJ or UVJ obstruction), or pathology that compresses the ureter from outside the ureter (enlarged lymph nodes for example).

**renal pelvis** - the central hollow area of the kidney where urine collects before it is transported to the ureter.

**renin** - an enzyme made and stored in the kidney that is important in blood pressure control.

**retrograde pyelogram** - an x-ray study in which radiopaque contrast is injected into the ureter from the bladder into the kidney collecting system. Usually done as in conjunction with cystoscopy.

**retroperitoneum** - the space behind the abdominal cavity (peritoneum) that contains large arteries and veins (aorta and vena cava), lymph nodes, kidneys, adrenal glands, pancreas.

**robotic surgery** - In urology, surgery done by attaching laparoscopic instruments and a camera to multiple robotic arms that are controlled by a surgeon sitting at a console.

**saw palmetto** - a natural supplement used to treat lower urinary tract symptoms cause by prostate enlargement. It comes from the fruit of the Serenoa repens tree.

**seminal vesicle** - a pair of glands that empty into the prostate via the ejaculatory ducts after joining with each vas deferens. 95% of the ejaculate comes from the semen made in the seminal vesicles.

**sepsis** - a consequence of a life -threatening infection in which the body's immune system response damages tissue and organs.

**septic shock** - a result of severe sepsis in which there is loss of blood pressure.

**serosa** - the outer membrane that covers organs of the body like the urinary bladder.

**shared decision making** - an exchange between patients and doctors working together to make decisions regarding tests, treatments, and care plans. The discussions involve weighing risks and benefits of treatments based on evidence and possible outcomes. Patient values, lifestyles, and expectations are discussed.

**skeletal muscle** - also known as striated muscle, attached to the bony skeleton and contracts in response to volitional nerve stimulation.

**smooth muscle** - muscle that occurs in internal organs not under voluntary control.

**staghorn calculus** - a large branched kidney stone that is often associated with an infection. A struvite stone can be a staghorn calculus and is made up of ammonium, phosphate, and magnesium. Also known as 'triple phosphate' stone.

**steroid** - organic compounds that include certain manufactured drugs, natural occurring hormones, and vitamins.

**stoma, catheterizable stoma** - a hollow organ like a segment of intestine that is usually attached to the skin. If one needs to place a catheter through the stoma to empty the contents of whatever needs to be transferred out of the body, it's called a catherizable stoma.

**stomal therapist** - a nurse who is an expert at taking care of stomas, the skin surrounding the stoma, and the appliances (drainage bags) that are sometimes necessary to collect bodily contents.

**testosterone** - male steroid hormone responsible for libido, sexual function, and male sexual characteristics.

**transitional cells** - type of cells that line the urinary bladder, ureter, and hollow collecting unit of the kidney (renal pelvis and calyces).

**transitional cell cancer** - also known as urothelial cell cancer, most common type of cancer of the bladder, ureter, internal portion of the kidney.

**tumor** - an abnormal mass or swelling of body tissue that can be benign or malignant.

**tumor markers in urine (NMP-22, FISH)** - proteins produced by cancer cells that can be measured in urine or blood. NMP stands for nuclear matrix protein, and FISH stands for fluorescence in situ hybridisation, and is a measure of genetic changes in DNA of tumors. Both of these tests are used to detect bladder cancer.

**tunica albuginea** - the dense tissue that encapsulates each spongy body (corpora cavernosa) of the penis (see Peyronie's Disease).

**TVO procedure** - a type of urethral sling procedure that places tension free urethral tape at slightly different exit incisions.

**TVT procedure/tension-free vaginal tape** - a procedure designed to provide support for the urethra so that when a cough or laugh or other increase of abdominal pressure occurs, the sphincters are in a position to work properly, and no leak occurs.

**ultrasound** - a painless imaging technique that that uses sound waves and involves no contrast and no x-rays. The sound waves create a picture called a sonogram of structures and organs in the body.

**UPJ** - ureteropelvic junction. Where the hollow internal part of the kidney called the renal pelvis joins the first part of the ureter (closest to the head).

**UVJ** - ureterovesical junction. Where the end of the ureter joins and empties into the bladder.

**ureter** - the straw-like hollow tube measuring about a foot in length that drains urine from the kidney into the bladder.

**ureteral orifice** - the end of the ureter as it ends in the bladder. On the floor of the bladder is a triangular shaped structure called the trigone. Each ureteral orifice is seen as a tiny hole and is the entrance to the ureter located at 2 of the 3 corners of the triangle.

**ureteroscope** - a fiber optic instrument with a camera on the end to allow an image to be displayed on a TV monitor. Usually flexible (but occasionally rigid), it has two working channels, one for saline, and the other for instruments like stone baskets or forceps.

**ureteroscopic lithotripsy** - a procedure that breaks up stones under direct vision using ureteroscope.

**urethra** - the tube through which the bladder drains urine.

**urethral meatus** - The hole at the end of the urethra - on the end of the penis in males, and top part of the vagina in females.

**urethral stricture** - a narrowing or scar within the urethra. A stricture can be very short (1-2 mm) or very long (> 2-3 cm).

**uric acid** - a breakdown product of purines responsible for stones of the same name and gout. Purines are found in a variety of foods (beans, peas, beer, liver, anchovies) and is a normal metabolite in the body.

**urine cytology** - a way of detecting cancer from the lining of the kidney, ureter, or bladder in which the cells are prepared in a special way and examined by the pathologist under the microscope.

**urobilinogen** - one of the chemicals routinely tested on  urinalysis that when positive can indicate liver disease.

**urgency** – a sudden desire to urinate.

**varicocoele** - a dilation of the veins in the scrotum that drain the testes, frequently described as a mass of varicose veins in the scrotum or "bag of worms."

**vas deferens/vas** – a thin tube about the diameter of a piece of spaghetti that carries sperm from the epididymis in the scrotum to the prostate where it meets the seminal vesicles to form the ejaculatory duct.

**virus** - a 'bug' that cannot be seen under standard light microscopy because it's too small and that consists of a segment of DNA or RNA and a protein coat that is able to cause an infection by multiplying only within living cells of a host.

# APPENDIX II

# References and Sources

## Introduction

Grad, Roland, et al. "Shared Decision Making in Preventative Medicine." PubMed Central, Canadian Fam Physician, 2017, Sept; 63(9): 682-684 < https://www.ncbi.nlm.nih.gov/pmc/articles/PMC5597010/

Elwyn, Gllyn, et al. "Shared Decision Making in Clinical Practice." J Gen Intern Med. 2012 Oct;27(10): 1361-1376 < https://www.ncbi.nlm.nih.gov/pmc/articles/PMC3445676/

## Chapter 1 - Human Plumbing

Kelly, Christopher and Landman, Jaimie. "The Netter Collection of Medical Illustrations: Urinary System. Vol. 5, 2nd Edition. Elsevier. Feb 21, 2012.

## Chapter 2 - I'm Peeing Blood

Loo RK, Lieberman SF, Slezak JM et al: Stratifying risk of urinary tract malignant tumors in patients with asymptomatic microscopic hematuria. Mayo Clin Proc 2013; 88:129.

Barocas, Daniel, et al. Microhematuria: AUA/SUFU Guideline 2020, Journal of Urology Oct 1, 2020; 778-786 < https://www.auajournals.org/doi/10.1097/JU.0000000000001297

# Chapter 3 - Incontinence, Overactive Bladder, Interstitial Cystitis

Kaiser Permanente Healthwise Staff, Seifert, Avery, urologist reviewer. Bladder Stress Test and Bonney Test for Urinary Incontinence in Women. Nov 8, 2019 < https://wa.kaiserpermanente.org/kbase/topic.jhtml?docId=hw219414

Rovner ES, Wein AJ: Treatment Options for Stress Urinary Incontinence. Rev Urol 2004; 6 (Suppl 3): S29-S47 < https://www.ncbi.nlm.nih.gov/pmc/articles/PMC1472859

Informed health.org (internet): Surgery for Pelvic Organ Prolapse. Aug 23, 2018 < https://www.ncbi.nlm.nih.gov/books/NBK525780/

Lightner DJ, et al: Diagnosis and treatment of overactive bladder (non-neurogenic) in adults" AUA/SUFU Guideline amendment 2019. J Urol 2019; 202: 558.

GormleyEA, et al: Diagnosis and treatment of overactive bladder (non-neurogenic) in adults: AUA/SUFU guideline. J Urol 2012; 188:2455

Cooperberg MR and Stoller ML (2005). "Percutaneous neuromodulation." *Urol Clin North Am* **32** (1): 71-8.

Ha Tanya and Xu Jue Hua: Interstitial cystitis intravesical therapy. Transl Androl Urol. 2017 Jul: 6(Suppl 2): S171-S179 <https://www.ncbi.nlm.nih.gov/pmc/articles/PMC5522791/

## Chapter 4 - Urinary Tract Infections

Anger J, et. al. Recurrent Uncomplicated Urinary Tract Infections in Women: AUA/CUA/SUFU Guideline, J Urol 2019; vol 202: 282-289

Valiquette L, Urinary tract infections in women. Can J Urol 2001 Jun; 8 Suppl 1: 6-12 <https://pubmed.ncbi.nlm.nih.gov/11442991/

Kovacs JS, Urinary Tract Infections (UTIs). WebMD 2021< https://www.webmd.com/women/guide/your-guide-urinary-tract-infections.

## Chapter 5 - Everybody Must Get Stones

Assimos D, Krambeck A, Miller NL et al: Surgical management of stones: American Urological Association/Endourological Society Guideline, part II. J Urol 2016; 196: 1161 >https://www.auanet.org/guidelines-and-quality/guidelines/kidney-stones-surgical-management-guideline.

Pearl, MS, et. al. Medical Management of Kidney Stones:     AUA Guideline. J. Urol. Aug 2014 <https://doi.org/10.1016/j.juro.2014.05.006

Hughes T, et. al. Guideline of guidelines for kidney and bladder stones. Turk J Urol. 2020 Nov; 46(Suppl1): S104-S112. <https://turkishjournalofurology.com/en/guideline-of-guidelines-for-kidney-and-bladder-stones

## Chapter 6 - Bladder Cancer

Chang, SS, et al. Treatment of Non-Metastatic Muscle Invasive Bladder Cancer: AUA/ASCO/ASTRO/SUO Guideline. J of Urol. 2017; 198: 552. amended 2020.

Chang, SS, et. al. Diagnosis and Treatment of Non-Muscle Invasive Bladder Cancer: AUA/SUO Guideline (2020) J Urol. 2016; 196: 1021.

Chu, C. et al (2021) "Use of Cxbladder Monitor during the COVID-19 Pandemic to reduce the frequency of surveillance cystoscopy" *The Journal of Urology 206* (3):1142e

Daneshmand S, Bartsch G. Improving selection of appropriate urinary diversion following radical cystectomy for bladder cancer. Expert Rev Anticancer Ther. 2011 Jun;11(6):941-8. doi: 10.1586/era.11.19. PMID: 21707291.

Daneshmand, S. et al. (2018) "Efficacy and Safety of Blue Light Flexible Cystoscopy with Hexaminolevulinate in the Surveillance of Bladder Cancer: A Phase III, Comparative, Multicenter Study" *The Journal of Urology 195* (5):1158-1165

## Chapter 7 - Renal Masses

Sigmon, DF, et. al. Renal Cyst. NIH, National Library of Medicine. May 2022 < https://www.ncbi.nlm.nih.gov/books/NBK470390/

Campbell, S, et. al. Renal Mass and Localized Renal Cancer: AUA Guideline. J Urol Sept 2017 < https://doi.org/10.1016/j.juro.2017.04.100

Wolf JS, Evaluation and Management of Solid Renal Masses: J of Urol, April 1998: Vol 159, pp 1120 -1133

Bamias, A, Current Clinical Practice Guidelines for the Treatment of Renal Cell Carcinoma: A Sestemativ Review and Critical Evaluation, Oncologist. 2017 Jun; 22(6): 667-697 <https://www.ncbi.nlm.nih.gov/pmc/articles/PMC5469586/

## Chapter 8 - Emergencies and Trauma

Morey AF, et. al. Urotrauma 2020: AUA Guideline. J Urol Jan 2021; vol 205 (1): 30-35.

# INDEX

## A

abdominal cavity, 162
adenocarcinoma, 105, 129, 147, 161
adjuvant, 114, 147
adrenal, 1, 10, 12, 132, 147, 162
adrenaline, 12, 147
adult polycystic, 148
alpha blocker, 148
anastomosis, 148
anatrophic nephrolithotomy, 92, 148
anterior repair, 45, 149
anticholinergics, 50
antidepressants, 54
aorta, 12, 162
arteriole, 149
artery, 149
asymptomatic, 21, 22, 23, 24, 26, 33,
    75, 148, 149, 167
atrophy, 48, 149

## B

bacteria, 20, 56, 59, 60, 61, 62, 63, 64,
    65, 66, 67, 68, 69, 77, 95, 111, 149,
    154, 155
bacteriuria, 5, 65, 149
benign, 6, 33, 64, 104, 124, 125, 127,
    129, 130, 131, 134, 148, 149, 164
bilirubin, 20, 150

bladder, 1, 5, 6, 10, 12, 14, 15, 19, 21,
    22, 27, 28, 29, 30, 31, 33, 35, 36,
    37, 38, 39, 40, 41, 42, 43, 44, 45,
    46, 47, 48, 49, 50, 51, 52, 53, 54,
    55, 56, 57, 59, 61, 62, 63, 64, 65,
    68, 69, 70, 71, 74, 75, 76, 78, 80,
    82, 84, 85, 86, 101, 103, 104, 105,
    106, 107, 108, 109, 110, 111, 112,
    113, 114, 116, 117, 118, 121, 131,
    137, 139, 141, 144, 145, 148, 149,
    150, 151, 152, 153, 155, 156, 157,
    158, 159, 160, 161, 162, 163, 164,
    165, 166, 168, 169, 170
bladder dysfunction, 40, 48
Blue Light Cystoscopy, 112
BUN, 149

## C

calcium oxalate, 83, 95, 96, 97, 98,
    99, 100, 150, 159
calculus, 150, 163
cancer, 4, 5, 6, 10, 12, 21, 22, 23, 24,
    25, 27, 29, 33, 52, 53, 56, 64, 103,
    104, 105, 107, 108, 109, 110, 111,
    112, 113, 114, 115, 116, 117, 121,
    123, 124, 126, 129, 130, 131, 132,
    133, 134, 135, 143, 144, 147, 149,
    150, 151, 156, 157, 158, 159, 161,
    164, 166,170

Cancer, 6, 103, 108, 169, 170
carcinoma in situ, 110, 150
CBC, 150
cells, 10, 11, 13, 20, 21, 67, 77, 103,
    104, 105, 107, 108, 110, 111, 131,
    150, 151, 153, 157, 158, 164, 166
chemotherapy, 110, 111, 114, 131,
    134, 147, 150, 151, 156, 158
citrate, 83, 97, 101, 151
creatinine, 101, 151
cryoablation, 124, 134, 151
cryotherapy, 157
CT scan, 24, 25, 27, 30, 31, 81, 84,
    93, 105, 124, 137, 139, 148, 151
CT urogram, 27, 30, 105, 151
Cxbladder, 112
cyst, 125, 126, 127, 152, 155
cystectomy, simple, 152
cystinuria, 152
cystitis, 5, 35, 52, 57, 61, 63, 66, 67,
    68, 69, 70, 71, 152, 156, 168
cystometrogram, 40, 49, 51, 152
cystoscope, 106
cystoscopy, 22, 23, 24, 25, 27, 29, 30,
    51, 53, 54, 71, 85, 106, 110, 152,
    162
Cystoscopy, 31, 32, 106

**D**

dihydrotestosterone, 152
disease, 4, 6, 33, 35, 48, 55, 62, 64,
    71, 96, 100, 109, 111, 112, 113,
    132, 148, 154, 157, 159, 161, 166
diverticulum, 63, 101, 153
doctor, 9, 18, 19, 26, 27, 30, 33, 40,
    41, 42, 47, 48, 53, 54, 56, 59, 60,
    61, 66, 68, 81, 107, 114, 133, 145,
    146, 159
double J stent, 86, 152
drugs., 49, 134

**E**

Elavil, 54
embolization, 153
emergencies, 4, 5, 6, 141
endoscope, 92, 153
endourology, 78, 153
erythropoietin, 13, 153
ESWL, 87, 88, 91, 102, 153, 158
external sphincter, 37, 38, 39, 42,
    118, 119, 154, 155

**F**

fallopian tubes, 114
Fesoterodine, 49
fever, 26, 60, 63, 64, 76, 77, 81, 90,
    127, 161
fluoroscopy, 79, 80, 87, 154
fungus, 59, 154

**G**

glands, 1, 10, 12, 147, 150, 158, 162
glans penis/clitoris, 154
glaucoma, 50
glucose, 13, 20, 154, 156
gross hematuria, 25, 29, 33

**H**

hematuria, 17, 19, 21, 22, 23, 24, 25,
    26, 27, 28, 29, 30, 33, 106, 154,
    167
hydrocele, 155

**I**

ileus, 76, 155
immune system, 67, 111, 147, 150,
    158, 162
Incontinence, 5, 35, 37, 43, 46, 168
infection, 16, 20, 27, 29, 33, 40, 44,
    47, 48, 49, 50, 57, 59, 61, 62, 63,

64, 65, 67, 68, 69, 70, 71, 77, 81, 86, 90, 91, 93, 95, 101, 104, 105, 111, 116, 120, 141, 149, 152, 155, 156, 161, 162, 163, 166

infections, 5, 15, 29, 52, 59, 60, 61, 62, 63, 64, 65, 68, 69, 70, 83, 95, 100, 115, 144, 169

inflammation, 53, 59, 65, 149, 152, 155, 161

internal sphincter, 38, 39, 44, 155

intra-vesical therapy, 156

**K**

Kaiser Permanente, 2, 143, 168

Kegel's exercises, 49, 54, 154

ketones, 20, 156

kidney, 4, 5, 6, 10, 14, 15, 19, 21, 23, 27, 29, 31, 33, 61, 63, 64, 65, 68, 70, 73, 74, 75, 76, 77, 80, 81, 82, 83, 84, 85, 88, 91, 92, 93, 94, 96, 108, 113, 123, 124, 125, 126, 127, 128, 129, 130, 131, 132, 133, 134, 135, 137, 139, 140, 141, 143, 144, 145, 146, 147, 148, 150, 151, 152, 153, 155, 158, 159, 160, 161, 162, 163, 164, 165, 166, 169

kidneys, 1, 5, 10, 11, 12, 13, 14, 27, 28, 29, 30, 31, 33, 59, 61, 63, 64, 68, 70, 71, 75, 78, 100, 103, 104, 107, 114, 117, 123, 124, 128, 148, 149, 151, 155, 156, 162

**L**

laparoscope, 156

laparoscopic, 115, 124, 126, 134, 156, 157, 162

leukocyte, 67, 156

lithotripsy, 74, 86, 88, 89, 102, 153, 156, 165

lumen, 14, 85, 157

*M*

malignant, 6, 107, 124, 125, 126, 129, 130, 131, 134, 135, 147, 150, 157, 164, 167

malignant., 125, 126, 129, 130, 134, 164

metastatic, 114, 124, 129, 131, 132, 134, 157

microscopic hematuria, 22

minimally invasive procedure, 91, 157

Mirabegron, 49, 50

MRI, 71, 95, 113, 124, 125, 129, 130, 132, 133, 155, 157

mucosa, 53, 103, 158

muscle, 12, 14, 42, 43, 47, 49, 50, 51, 52, 53, 55, 56, 80, 103, 108, 109, 110, 112, 113, 114, 115, 148, 154, 155, 157, 158, 159, 163

**N**

nausea, 63, 64, 76, 77, 81, 128, 161

neo-adjuvant, 147

neoadjuvant therapy, 158

neobladder, 55, 117, 118, 119, 120, 158, 159

nephron, 13, 158

nephrostomy tube, 91, 92, 141, 158

nerves, 36, 47, 48, 49, 51, 52, 159

neurotransmitter, 158

**O**

oncologist, 113, 121, 132, 134, 135, 159, 161

osteoporosis, 159

Overactive Bladder, 5, 35, 46, 168

oxalate, 95, 97, 98, 99, 100, 150, 159

Oxybutynin, 49

**P**

painful, 32, 53, 54, 57, 66, 85, 102, 148
partial nephrectomy, 126, 159
PCP, 18, 19, 24, 47, 49, 50, 51, 60, 71, 145, 160
penis, 154, 159, 164, 165
perineum, 160
peritoneal cavity, 160
pH, 20, 67, 101, 160
Physician, 160, 167
placebo, 160
posterior repair, 45, 160
psychogenic impotence, 160
pyelolithotomy, 92, 161
pyelonephritis, 5, 63, 65, 77, 161
pyridium, 54

**R**

radiation therapy, 64, 161
re-canalization, 161
renal colic, 6, 76, 161
renal pelvis, 65, 80, 84, 92, 93, 148, 161, 162, 164, 165
renin, 13, 162
retrograde pyelogram, 162
retroperitoneum, 11, 27, 129, 162
robotic, 124, 134, 135, 157, 162

**S**

seminal vesicle, 162
sepsis, 61, 64, 77, 91, 162
septic, 77, 90, 162
serosa, 53, 103, 163
shared decision making, 2, 3, 7, 8, 88, 143, 163
skeletal, 103, 154, 155, 163
Solifenacin, 49
steroid, 163, 164

stoma, 116, 117, 155, 163
stomal therapist, 116, 163
stones, 4, 5, 6, 10, 27, 32, 33, 63, 65, 73, 74, 75, 76, 77, 78, 79, 80, 81, 83, 84, 88, 91, 92, 93, 94, 95, 96, 97, 98, 99, 100, 101, 102, 140, 143, 144, 148, 152, 153, 156, 159, 160, 161, 165, 166, 169
surgery, 2, 4, 40, 41, 43, 44, 45, 55, 114, 115, 121, 126, 130, 131, 132, 133, 135, 138, 139, 141, 144, 147, 155, 156, 157, 158, 159, 162

**T**

testosterone, 152, 164
Tolterodine (Detrol), 49
trauma, 5, 7, 137, 138
treatment, 2, 3, 4, 5, 6, 7, 10, 15, 17, 33, 49, 51, 52, 54, 55, 56, 59, 61, 64, 71, 74, 77, 78, 79, 81, 101, 102, 110, 111, 113, 124, 125, 129, 130, 131, 132, 133, 134, 135, 144, 146, 147, 151, 158, 159, 160, 161, 168
Trospium, 49
tumor, 6, 31, 33, 104, 105, 106, 107, 108, 109, 112, 115, 123, 124, 129, 130, 132, 133, 134, 135, 145, 150, 152, 157, 158, 159, 161, 164
Tumor, 106
tunica albuginea, 164
TVO procedure, 164

**U**

ultrasound, 30, 40, 48, 54, 64, 68, 70, 71, 80, 81, 91, 92, 93, 95, 101, 124, 125, 153, 155, 160, 164
ureter, 1, 10, 14, 63, 64, 65, 76, 80, 84, 85, 86, 88, 91, 92, 103, 117, 120, 141, 148, 150, 152, 153, 158, 161, 162, 164, 165, 166

ureteroscope, 86, 88, 89, 91, 165

ureteroscopy, 88, 91

urethra, 1, 10, 12, 14, 15, 19, 21, 31, 32, 38, 39, 41, 42, 43, 44, 59, 61, 62, 63, 65, 66, 68, 69, 70, 71, 86, 101, 104, 106, 115, 117, 118, 119, 120, 137, 139, 141, 148, 150, 152, 154, 155, 158, 159, 164, 165, 166

urethral stricture, 62, 166

urgency, 21, 26, 27, 35, 36, 45, 53, 60, 166

uric acid, 77, 81, 95, 96, 101, 166

urinary retention, 44, 54, 56

urine, 5, 6, 11, 13, 14, 15, 17, 18, 19, 20, 21, 22, 23, 25, 26, 27, 28, 29, 30, 32, 33, 35, 36, 37, 38, 39, 40, 47, 49, 50, 52, 53, 55, 59, 60, 61, 62, 63, 64, 65, 66, 67, 68, 70, 71, 75, 76, 77, 79, 80, 81, 82, 91, 96, 97, 98, 100, 101, 103, 104, 105, 107, 109, 117, 118, 119, 120, 124, 127, 138, 139, 143, 145, 146, 149, 151, 152, 154, 155, 156, 158, 159, 160, 161, 162, 164, 165, 166

urobilinogen, 20, 166

urologist, 9, 17, 18, 20, 21, 24, 26, 27, 28, 29, 30, 31, 36, 40, 43, 47, 48, 49, 50, 51, 54, 56, 59, 62, 71, 73, 79, 81, 82, 84, 86, 88, 90, 92, 93, 94, 95, 101, 102, 105, 106, 107, 108, 111, 113, 120, 121, 125, 129, 130, 131, 132, 134, 135, 139, 141, 144, 152, 168, 178

urology, 1, 2, 8, 24, 78, 143, 144, 145, 148, 151, 153, 162

uterus, 12, 27, 29, 45, 114, 152

UTI, 4, 5, 6, 18, 27, 33, 48, 53, 59, 60, 61, 62, 65, 66, 67, 68, 69, 70, 71

**V**

vagina, 29, 41, 42, 43, 45, 62, 66, 105, 114, 116, 141, 152, 160, 165

varicocoele, 166

virus, 59, 155, 166

# ACKNOWLEDGEMENTS

This book took eight years to write. I relied on professional writers, teachers, colleagues, and friends to help with this process. Without their encouragement and expertise, there would still be a disorganized mess of a file on my laptop. It is here that I would like to express my heartfelt gratitude to: Dr. Janice Harper, superb copywriter and editor, Dr. Roger Porter, English professor, author, food critic, and friend, Martin Stabler; the late Luis Halpert, M.D., John Barry, M.D., Rich Steinberg, M.D., Ron Loo, M.D., Jerry Slepack, M.D., Steven Skoog, M.D., P.J. Chandhoke, M.D., Doug Ackerman, M.D., Jeffrey Johnson, M.D., Patrick Maginn, M.D., Eugene Fuchs, M.D., the late Thomas Hatch, M.D., Roger Wicklund, M.D., Adriene Carmack, M.D., Craig Sadur, M.D., Thomas Kelsey, M.D., Matt Forsyth, M.D., Richard Burt, M.D., Matti Totonchy, M.D., Bruce Lowe, M.D., Ron Potts, M.D., Jill Einstein, M.D., Barbara Loeb, M.D., LoAn Nguyen, M.D., Kieth Bachman, M.D., Christopher Nelson, M.D., Anita Nelson, Steve Williams, M.D., Violeta Rabrinovitch, Tim Carey, M.D., Avery Seifert, M.D., Tracy Sanford, John Scott, and Lyman Flayhive, and all of the M.A.V.E.N. Project volunteer specialists who provide specialty consultation to primary care providers and patients in over 200 free clinics in 19 U.S. States. I would also like to thank the over 50 Oregon Health Science University residents whom I had the honor of sharing the joys of being a urologist with for 31 years. And, I thank my brother Lenny Lieberman, and sister Sherry Preiss.

Finally, special thanks to my wife Virginia, and my daughters Emily Karlberg (Lieberman), and Elizabeth Lieberman, M.D., who provided unconditional support throughout the eight years I worked on researching and writing this book.

www.ingramcontent.com/pod-product-compliance
Lightning Source LLC
Chambersburg PA
CBHW071036050426

42335CB00051B/2108